## Stay young for ever

If you talk to Eileen Fowler about her career, she says, 'Well, presentation is my middle name and from the beginning I realized that if I wanted to persuade people to do exercises, they must be presented attractively.' Eileen found the way to do this by spending ten years in the theatre, appearing in musical comedy, plays and cabaret in London and the provinces. Combining physical education with theatrical presentation, she started a Keep Fit class in her local village during 1934. It was an immediate success and within five years she controlled an industrial Keep Fit organization in three counties.

The war years were spent in Hertfordshire, training and teaching war workers in offices and factories in Welwyn Garden City. Eileen married in 1945 but began teaching again and by 1954 was demonstrating her exercises on television in B.B.C. women's programmes. Three years later her own programme was launched with a team of Birmingham Keep Fit housewives, and it ran until 1961.

Then came B.B.C. radio *Woman's Hour* and six months as a guest of the West of England Players at B.B.C. Bristol. After a television series in 1963, she began in 1964 her country-wide tours teaching Keep Fit exercises to thousands of women. During this time she was broadcasting in *Woman's Hour* a 'Stay Young' series. In 1971 she joined the *Today* programme, teaching family Keep Fit every morning during the week at ten minutes to seven, and she is currently appearing on B.B.C. 1.

In the New Year Honours List she was awarded the M.B.E.

**Eileen Fowler**

# Stay young for ever

**Pan Books Ltd**
London and Sydney

First published 1963 by George Newnes Ltd
This revised edition published 1975 by
Pan Books Ltd, Cavaye Place, London SW10 9PG
ISBN 0 330 24471 X


A number of the Keep Fit diagrams in this book are based on original drawings by Jack Dunkley previously published by B.B.C. Publications, to both of whom author and publisher extend their acknowledgements and thanks

Printed in Great Britain by
Hazell Watson & Viney Ltd, Aylesbury, Bucks

# Contents

# Preface

Barbara Cartland

This book is as gay, invigorating and exciting as Eileen Fowler herself.

I shall never forget the day she first came to see me. She walked into my home like a small, radiant ray of sunshine. She positively glowed with health and at the same time there was something sweet, gentle and sympathetic about her that I found irresistible. I soon discovered what it was.

Eileen, like myself, believes that she must help people. It is not money, being a personality, or power which makes her work so hard, which gives her the energy to write books like this on top of her overwhelmingly busy schedule.

It is all a pattern and a design for helping other people not as lovely and as well as herself.

I know nothing more satisfying than to help someone to health, because good health is the foundation of everything we do and are. Eileen does this with her exercises, not only because they give women a good figure like her own, but because they do so much more.

Her exercises produce beauty and grace in the mind as well as the body. They are worked out to bring also peace and serenity, relaxation and rhythm. All these things are essentials to women living in the bustling, tempestuous, crisis-prone world of today.

I am willing to bet that none of Eileen's regular pupils has ever had a nervous breakdown, and I am convinced every time I see them that their husbands or their husbands-to-be are exceptionally lucky men because they are almost assured a happy marriage.

Need I say more, except read this book? It is full of the magic that only Eileen Fowler can give us.

Bless her.

B.C.

# Introduction

Hello! Here I am in the garden as usual – or, to be exact, in my studio. I always come here to think. I am happiest in the fresh air. I love the house, too; it's on the top of a hill right in the middle of an Essex village. The old archway and courtyard are much the same as they were several hundred years ago, but Keep Fit is a young and vital way of life and more at home in the studio. It wasn't always a studio, but now it's very light, with big glass doors and a partly glazed roof. My favourite marigolds fill the flower beds and the River Thames is just visible in the distance. Here I can practise my exercises in rain or shine. So it's natural that I should come here to write my first book, which I hope you will find useful. These are the ways I have found to stay young.

**My way of life**

Not long ago I celebrated my twentieth anniversary on television and sound radio. I'll never forget the date. It was April 1st, 1954. With a mischievous look, my mother had said, 'What a curious day to start, dear. I hope you don't make a fool of yourself.'

There were ten thousand letters after that first afternoon broadcast and the exercise leaflets that went out all over the country were the forerunners of supplements and charts in the *Radio Times* and an unbroken series of Keep Fit programmes on B.B.C. Television.

I love getting the letters – so does my husband; he often helps me with a knotty problem which needs a very personal answer. They come from all over the world, forging links with friends I never see. It's lovely to hear of an Eileen

Fowler Class in New Zealand, Bombay or South Africa and I long, at times, to visit them. . . .

The first Eileen Fowler Class started in a village years ago when I left the Stage. The theatre was my first love. 'Presentation' has always been my middle name. It's so important. Whether it's a show, a dress or a meal – however simple – it must be put on properly. I learnt about this from producers who really love their job, and I learnt about staying young from the artistes. Many of them were years older than me, but they were vital, full of fun, and had such perfect poise.

One Scottish woman in particular was very lovely at sixty, with a slender figure and beautiful complexion. She told me that fresh air was the secret. 'It feeds me,' she said, 'keeps me young, and of course I keep to a light diet and I exercise daily.'

Bit by bit it dawned on me that it was not necessary to age as fast as many women I knew. My French grandmother, with her slender *chic*, had told me that as you mature your figure and your feet become more important than your face, that good posture and quick movements give a youthful appearance in later life. Before I realized it I was caught up in this fascinating hobby – how to stay young. But I soon wanted more. I wanted to study and to teach. So I left the theatre and started on a new career.

Exercise was to be the basis of my work; keeping all the muscles toned up so that they remain firm and prevent the figure from sagging and thickening. 'Keep Fit' – that was it – with a strong beauty angle.

Which reminds me that my first introduction to Keep Fit as we understand it today was a peal of laughter from Miss Kay Evans, senior technical adviser to the Central Council of Physical Recreation, when I demonstrated a trunk exercise to her.

I was standing in her office one afternoon in 1934, rather flushed and a tiny bit self-conscious, explaining quite seriously that I characterized my exercises and that I was meant to be Sir Walter Raleigh. The simple downward movement was to place the cloak before Queen Elizabeth the First and then I would uncurl slowly, drawing myself up to full height, feeling very tall.

How she laughed! I was humming a suitable Tudor tune at the time. I went on to explain in as dignified a manner as possible that I had been trained from childhood to move, but when I had to choose between gymnastics and the theatre (my other love and my life for the previous ten years) I chose the latter. In spite of this, for many years I still had a yearning to teach all the time that I was appearing in musical comedy. In fact, I often used to get some rather reluctant but kind-hearted members of the cast to join me on a darkened stage some mornings doing bending, twisting and stretching exercises for the good of their figures. Now, I explained solemnly to Miss Evans, I was preparing to break with the theatre and take up Keep Fit. I wanted to teach it the right way, the sensible, attractive way that could make it part of every woman's daily round, rather than the separate almost cranky thing that some people considered it in those days before the war.

My demonstration, given in good faith and performed quite seriously, had caused a moment of amusement. Even so, I was not far wrong in basing my little 'pantomime' on the courtly sweeping movements of an Elizabethan courtier, for one thing we always teach in Keep Fit is wide, graceful movement, generous and without rigidity. The days of 'physical jerks' are long over. Jerky exercises can even do more damage than good.

To me Keep Fit became more than an exercise routine to be done in a weekly class, or practised at home. It became a way of living, but never in any sense a cult – just a down-to-earth, practical and natural, sensible way to stay young and enjoy life to the full. Staying young is not just a matter of keeping the wrinkles and the grey hair at bay.

Modern make-up and hairdressing, though they work miracles, do not hide the tension in your face when you are exhausted, or the frown lines in your forehead caused by backache and tired feet; but a knowledge of movement *will*. Healthy, toned-up muscles and a body trained to take the onslaught of time will get you through your most exacting day. In this age of jets, jazz, and keeping up with the Joneses, it's all too easy for a woman to lose her way and race dizzily against the clock through the demanding routine of the day, unaware of the toll it is taking.

Have you ever stopped and watched the passers-by in a busy street? I often do, and nine out of ten women's faces wear a tense and harassed look – even if they are out shopping for something pretty to wear. I often wonder whether they've suddenly caught sight of themselves in a long mirror and been disappointed at their reflection. Time and again I've done this and made myself slow up, made myself smile to prevent all the lines of my face from running down. And I take a very firm hold of myself, too, when trying on anything in a fitting-room with strip lighting. It's most misleading – makes me look a hundred!

I know that half a lifetime given to a family can leave precious little time to devote to one's own youth and beauty. I believe that the average woman's life is extremely unselfish and my heart aches when I see somebody's mother becoming over-exhausted and giving away her birthright as a woman – her right to stay young, to stay vital and attractive, not to wake up one day and wonder where her youthful good looks have gone, but to have the joy of them all her life.

My friends always laugh when I say, 'We owe it to ourselves

to look good and feel good' – and so we do, for our family's sake as well as our own.

'Tuesday's child is full of grace.' I love that old saying, but why can't we be Saturday's child – 'Work hard for a living' – and still have Tuesday's grace?

Of course we can, and we will.

# General information

*All enquiries* to Eileen Fowler, High House, Horndon-on-the-Hill, Essex.

**Keeping fit at home**

Exercises for everyone, pages 61 to 92, will teach the basic movements. The sequences at the end of the book, pages 93 to 96, can be practised to suitable tunes on the radio or recordings with a steady beat and tempo. Several recordings have been made of exercises taught during television and sound radio programmes. See 'Keep Fit Records', below. When using these records it is advisable to break down the movements and learn them carefully before doing them up to tempo with the music.

These records have been used all over the country to start up groups, particularly in rural districts where it is not possible to obtain an experienced Leader or pianist.

A special Keep Fit Day is organized in London at regular intervals for those wishing to teach television Keep Fit. See 'Keep Fit with Eileen Fowler', below.

When starting a private class amongst friends or fellow-workers it is important to have a room with a stage so that the Leader can easily be seen by every member of the class.

A good floor is necessary for exercises taken sitting or lying down. Soft slippers are usually worn, and stretch slacks with jersey top, tights and leotard, or a Keep Fit tunic are all suitable for this type of movement.

If a pianist is not available, a selection of instrumental

records is helpful for class 'breaks' and activities, these to be used to vary the class programme and in addition to special Keep Fit recordings.

*1. 'Keep Fit with Eileen Fowler'*, a Keep Fit day course for teachers, Leaders and potential Leaders, is held twice a year in London during the spring and autumn.

*2. 'Meet Eileen Fowler' Rallies* are arranged from time to time throughout the country.

*3. Keep Fit Records*
Family Keep Fit (in stereo) REC 174
Slim to Rhythm (in stereo) REC 132
Stay Young (in mono) REC 18

At the piano – Helen Shields
Electric organ – Roy Cloughton
Drums – Ray Smith

All records carry a B.B.C. label and are available from Boosey & Hawkes, Upper Regent St., London W.1., and good record dealers.

*4. New Cassette* – 'Stay Slim with Eileen Fowler'. A top selection from her Keep Fit recordings.

*5. Eileen Fowler Keep Fit Badges*
Full particulars of *Leadership Training* and local classes can be obtained from The Keep Fit Association, 70 Brompton Road, London SW3 1HE.

*6.* For *Keep Fit Classes* run by your Education Authority, apply to the local Education Office.

*7.* Particulars of *Coaching Holidays* in a variety of indoor and outdoor activities, including golf, tennis and swimming are obtainable from The Sports Council, 70 Brompton Road, London SW3 1HE.

# How to practise

Learn the Basic Movements one by one – as you would the notes of a piano. In this way you can build up a series of Keep Fit exercises which can be done easily and well. Pages 93–96 show basic movements linked together to form sequences and placed to give some degree of balance. First, a warm-up, using arms and shoulders; followed by a hip exercise; then a tummy sequence and a final whole body movement. In this way no groups of muscles are used for too long at a time. When linking basic movements to form new sequences, each one should flow into the other with relaxed continuity. Music should be steady or slow for big movements, and light and catchy for smaller ones, i.e. a hand, foot or shoulder shrug. A tuneful chorus of 32 bars can be used for a simple sequence, giving time for an energetic movement, and a more restful one, and using 8 or 16 bars for each, as required.

**Terms of movement**

Beat – to slap with palm of hand.
Snap Fingers – to click thumb and third finger.
Sweep – to make a continuous and extending curving movement.
Bounce – an easy bending of the knees more than once.

# 1 The five golden keys

Here they are; the Five Golden Keys to staying young. They have a familiar ring but they work as well today as they did when our mothers first handed them down to us. *Exercise, Fresh Air, Sensible Eating, Relaxation, and Enough Sleep.*

Following these rules doesn't mean that you cannot smoke or drink in moderation, or that you have to swallow vitamin pills by the hundred, or become a food crank. On the contrary, they help you to enjoy life, not make you suffer.

Let's take daily exercise first.

The look of horror on some people's faces when I mention exercise always amuses me. 'I can touch my toes,' they say, 'without bending my knees, too! So please don't make me do anything else.'

'But it's fun,' I tell them, 'wonderful fun, and I want you to bend your knees.'

It is fun, that is why it is the answer to most of our minor nervous and physical problems – but naturally women want to know how.

'How will exercise help me?' they say. 'Surely housework makes me move most of my muscles.' Even so a specially designed set of exercises will gradually train a way of movement that will help you to use your housework to benefit your figure and your health. It is the *way* you move that counts.

Constant upward stretching pulls your bust up and away

from your hips, leaving a flat, long midriff, which is the basis of a good figure. Don't let's worry too much yet about what is above and below the waistline. Let's make sure that we never, ever slump in the middle, that we pull upwards and away as often as possible, stretching with our arms way above our heads, not just placing them there but thinking about how the muscles of the midriff are stretching and toning up – then they will be able to hold you that way all of the time.

Like this we are helping to banish backache, too, because we are opening up the vertebrae of the spine. When we slump we are allowing the vertebrae to settle down on each other, preventing the blood from circulating freely and gradually building up tension and strain.

So lift the chest, stand tall, let the whole body fall into line.

Slumping thickens the waistline, gives the figure a square look and results in a spare tyre, which makes the perfect base for middle-age spread. It is not always overweight that makes us concerned about our lack of a flat tummy. Very often this is entirely due to the way we stand, simply because we have allowed back and tummy muscles, which work together, to become slack.

Exercise will put this right. Exercise will help to break down fatty deposits which build into bulges. It will fine down your figure. It will help to relax the too-thin and over-energetic who cannot store sufficient fat to give them the pretty curves they want. It is a health giver; a beautifier; a relaxer; and a *Must* for all women.

But let us suppose that you have a perfect figure already – then exercise will keep it that way. Let us suppose that you move with lissom, youthful grace. Will you always be able to do so? Are you sure that you will always have time for a swim, a round of golf, or a vigorous game of tennis? If not, then take up Keep Fit right away. Not for you the heaviness of later life, the nervous tension, the curious closing down of movement in neck, shoulders, hip and knee joints which affects so many women, and is so ageing.

Just as an acrobat or a dancer must limber up every day if her performance is not to suffer – so must you. Muscles moved insufficiently and joints left to stiffen deteriorate fast. Exercise is necessary to deepen the breathing, to take in more oxygen which cleanses the bloodstream.

These are some of the reasons for exercise, but what about the fun ? The fun is in moving to music, the exhilaration of moving in rhythm – any rhythm, all rhythm from classical to pop. The fun is in the relaxation which comes from doing modern Keep Fit, in the sense of achievement, in the social side, in the upsurge of energy and vitality. It is in the compliments on your looks and good temper, the fun of doing it at home on your own and surprising everyone, and never, never looking your age.

It is never too soon and never too late to begin preparing to stay young and attractive all your life. Whether you are just emerging from childhood, or whether it's a bit difficult to remember those days, it doesn't matter. The Five Golden Keys will help unlock the door to vitality and the joy of living.

Many Keep Fit Leaders are in my age-group, and they are living examples of what they teach. So are the thousands of woman all over the country who Keep Fit at home – sometimes on their own, or with a friend or neighbour who pops in for a cup of tea, an exercise and a chat. Women do not need a schedule for keeping fit. Any time is the right time, and anywhere the right place to do it – in the middle of the housework, in the bathroom, garden or kitchen. As long as you are comfortably dressed, you can swing and stretch and bend to your fullest capacity. If you've got the radio switched on it's easy. Sooner or later you will hear a tune with a definite beat, and you are away.

Some of the exercises in this book are 'do-it-yourself' ones so that when you have got the idea you can fit the movements to any rhythm. Then exercise becomes a natural – as much a part of your daily life as cleaning your teeth or brushing your hair. Why should so much time be spent on the face and so little on the figure? Don't let yours be the poor relation. Take care of it. Work to keep it slim and straight and supple as a reed.

Because of the way we bend our knees and relax as often as we stretch, an understanding of relaxation becomes part of ourselves. Sometimes I wonder whether, after all, this is not the most valuable part of Keeping Fit, because when you are relaxed, everything falls into place in your mind, and you are able to cope so much more easily with any problems you may have to face. A saner sense of values emerges and you realize that something you were so worried about is not perhaps quite so important after all, that you are not alone with your worries, that the power of good is frighteningly effective if you know how to harness it and don't insist on taking the reins yourself all of the time.

If you are tired, overwrought and tense, make yourself move to music – even a few minutes will help. Then take a break: feet up and a cup of something hot, but don't add the sticky bun or half a dozen biscuits. One of our Golden Keys fits the kind of larder that will slim you and not fatten you.

When you exercise, really move – not jerkily or timidly but smoothly, fluidly and to your fullest capacity. If you are reaching up to the ceiling, really try to touch it. If you are stretching to the wall of your room, bend your knees so that you can get farther over and try to get there. If you are dropping down towards the floor, relax and let yourself go.

Those of us who yearn to be taller need not dread loosing height as the years go by. This type of Keep Fit, with its emphasis on walking tall, does really keep your precious inches. One Leader of sixty-five used to be the shortest of the family of three sisters, but her work, she says, has made her the tallest now. Her sisters have, in fact, lost a little of their height by sinking into age, while she has retained hers by constantly standing, sitting and walking tall. She has retained her supple and slim figure because she loves to move to music and because she is conscious of the way she moves.

When you help your muscles to maintain their elasticity, you move with grace in a supple, youthful way, and the good work goes on. If you just let things take their course and make no effort, you may end up by moving in one piece – in a solid, ageing sort of way.

Keep moving. Keep young. A great deal of rheumatism could be kept at bay if only the joints all over the body were moved to music, every day. Fingers and hands, feet and ankles, knees and hips, and the neck which becomes stiff and tense so easily.

Anyone who sits all day in an office can benefit from becoming Keep Fit minded. Did you know that sitting still for hours can be very wearing? Movement is the antidote! You can sit and stay supple if you do the exercises in a chair which are shown between pages 79 and 84. I am going to do some now. My arm aches from writing!

The sun is shining, and I am still in my studio in the garden where I have learnt that gardening is grand for youth and beauty. I kneel as much as I can and save the old door mats for the job. Bending can be so tiring and so ugly if you keep your knees straight and your seat sticks out. It's so much more comfortable and prettier to bend your knees. When you pick up anything heavy, like a pile of seed boxes or a pail of water, get close to it and bend your knees, relax your shoulders, breathe in when you lift, making your legs bring you up. Don't let your back take all the strain. That goes for lifting the baby, too. Why cots have to be so low, I don't know. Try to keep your feet apart and knees easy. Or one foot in front of the other, bending down in a curtsy position is more relaxed, and less likely to make your back ache because you keep it straighter.

Many of our big-movement exercises bring in this type of relaxing and dropping down to the floor – very useful because you can get used to moving this way in everyday life. Swinging is good too. In Keep Fit we do a lot of that, often picking up a scarf, tea towel, brush or something weighing about two pounds. We swing it around in circles. It gives real freedom of movement, lifts the bust-line, and is wonderful for the circulation. We twist quite a bit for our waistline, but always with feet apart and an easy change of weight, by rocking from foot to foot. We bend our knees as in a golf swing, so that we can relax and get farther round. The days of jerky P.T. are mercifully over and now even a cat (my favourite animal) has nothing on us in the way of fluid movement.

So give exercise all you've got! Don't be stingy with little tentative movements, don't place your movements, swing into them with a confident air. Relax and enjoy yourself. Dance a bit too. Your feet and ankles will appreciate a little limbering up, and don't forget to relax and curl down to the floor, coming up slowly, head last, to your full height. This is for the sake of your spine, your figure, and for staying young.

# 2 Fresh air

'Good gracious! You haven't changed a bit.' After thirty-three years a remark like this can be music to the ears. It certainly was to mine on that occasion in the West Country when I was meeting friends after all that time.

We were remembering a wonderful bicycle made of Parma violets which had been handed up to me on the stage of the Princes Theatre, Bristol, on the last night of a pantomime in which I played Principal Boy. That Christmas we were having a great many matinées. This left little time to get out in the fresh air, but I had amused many people, and caused some publicity, by cycling all over the place in the mornings. I had to have fresh air! I knew that breakfast in bed and late rising would not help me to get through the exciting but tiring hours in the theatre; but fresh air did. I remembered the advice of a Scottish friend and got out whenever possible. At the end of the run, I was almost as fresh as when I started.

I still cycle for fresh air, I 'breathe' and I walk. Let's take this question of breathing first. When you get up in the morning open the window wide and let every scrap of air out of your lungs. Force it all out; then fill up slowly with fresh air; three times will be enough. It gives you a fresher feeling and lifts the chest – important for good posture. It can also help to break the habit of shallow breathing which does not give the lungs a chance to expand. We need oxygen to cleanse the bloodstream and to get rid of impurities in our system, to make the eyes bright and the cheeks glow and to bring a shine to the hair.

I love to walk. Not, I might say, clutching a handbag or

umbrella while teetering along on high heels; that I suffer only when I have to. A favourite mackintosh and comfortable shoes and I'm away. When my mind is full of problems out I go. Little by little I stop looking in; my introspection goes and I am noticing the trees, the birds in the country, or the hats, if I'm in town. Hundreds of muscles move in rhythm as I step out from the hips, chin up, a smug smile on my face because I know I am fining down my figure and improving the shape of my legs and ankles – and staying young.

Oh, for that wonderful tonic – a morning to oneself; a morning when we can slam the door on household cares and, if we are living in a town or suburb, there's time to take a bus to the nearest patch of green.

Sometimes I like to spend a day in the open air – just walking. Where? Anywhere. Perhaps I'll finish up at the cinema in the next town and see a film. I have as little time to waste as the next woman yet I feel that this cannot be regarded as a waste of time because I know the value of such things. I know that to do something that is a little crazy, that is young, that makes your husband and your friends laugh, achieves more for a woman's happiness and self-confidence than a mink coat.

Health is so often just a matter of habit. We must teach ourselves to lead the lives that make us healthy no matter what we may imagine others are thinking. Perhaps a young housewife living in a suburban street may not like the thought of facing the surprised stare of her neighbours or the slightly shocked look of friends when she admits she has been for a two-hour walk and left some of the chores unfinished!

How terrible that we can be so influenced by what other people think! We are, perhaps, not conscious of it. We think we lead the lives we want to lead but insidiously the opinions and ways and habits of other people leave their mark upon us and we are afraid of not conforming: it takes courage to be different.

Anyone worried about weight below the waistline should walk it off. When walking for health we should walk fairly fast – the faster we move, the faster we will lose weight.

Men walk better than women because their clothes give them hip freedom and they wear comfortable shoes. They usually stride out freely and hold themselves upright.

So start off on the right foot by making sure your girdle is not too long. If it grips the thighs you will probably have to toddle from the knees. If you walk regularly you will not need a heavy girdle anyway. Too much pressure is bad for the tops of the legs and can lead to varicose veins. If you get back-ache, walking will help you by strengthening the muscles which keep you upright and support your spine.

When you walk, push off with the back foot and keep your feet parallel and close together. If you think you bob about or roll from side to side, walk in slow motion for a few yards; this will show up any faults and make it easier to correct them. When wearing high heels it is essential not to stride; take smaller steps than normal.

Do not clutch your handbag under your arm with your shoulder hunched; and watch that shopping – two light bags are better than one heavy one. If you must use one only, change it frequently from hand to hand.

It is the opinion of the Arthritis and Rheumatic Council that women are more subject to rheumatic pains than men, largely because they are constantly placing an unnatural strain on their shoulder muscles through carrying heavy handbags and overloaded shopping baskets. Plenty of physical exercise and such games as tennis, using the arms, help to keep the muscles in trim. For heavy shopping, baskets on wheels are recommended to take the strain off the shoulder muscles.

Walk, then, without your handbag and shopping as often as you can in the fresh air. Come in glowing with exercise, having breathed oxygen for hours, head up, eyes alight and a picture of youth and beauty. These are the things which count, if you want to stay young for ever.

# 3 Sensible eating

'Foody Fowler' was my nickname at school and I still love to eat, but no more stodgy foods, fatty or fried. Oh dear, no! I've more respect for my figure, my skin and my energy. No more sticky buns and gooey cakes.

I would be the last to deny that it suits some women to be plump and rigid dieting would only take away their bonny looks; what a price to pay for losing an inch or two off their measurements! But a great many of us feel better and look better at the right weight for our height and age. I cannot talk about crash diets because I would not attempt to follow one without my doctor's permission. (I nearly did once and became so tired and irritable that the result was a food spree and a large collection of broken skirt zips!)

I've learnt my lesson and I eat sensibly. To keep down to the 8½ stone (54 kg.) my 5 ft. 3 in. demands, I find one really good meal a day is plenty, backed up of course by a light fruit breakfast, morning coffee, a light lunch and a cup of tea if I want it. I enjoy an occasional drink – especially in the evening when my husband comes home – alcoholic if I think I need it, or tomato juice if I don't.

To keep slim and youthful, exercise and sensible eating must go hand in hand. All the exercises in this book performed ten times a day won't work if combined with a big breakfast, a large lunch or dinner and a hot, tasty supper. However, the Keep Fit way of eating certainly doesn't leave you hungry. My meals are by no means small but they don't fill up every corner. Based mainly on the protein foods, my main meal – eaten sometimes at midday, sometimes at night – is always made up of meat, poultry, fish, eggs, bacon or ham, according to how I have planned my working day. When I am very busy, I don't always get as many green vegetables as I would like, but never by-pass my salad.

A friend of mine who insists she doesn't eat enough to keep a mouse alive, gained half a stone during her holiday. She was persuaded to try my method although she thought it would be rather slow. It was. It took eight weeks to lose eight pounds, but the weight has never returned. She is exercising every day and her clothes all fit beautifully once more. She is running upstairs instead of walking and says she feels on top of the world. She certainly looks it!

This is a case when a crash diet would have done the trick sooner but she would probably have ruined her looks. So often in extreme dieting, as the pounds fade away, the skin sags and wrinkles and the whole purpose is defeated. Age is the result, not youth. It is far better to form a habit of sensible eating that will last a lifetime and save the constant worry of watching the scales.

So much depends on our own individual metabolism. Those of us with a high metabolic rate tend to be slim, sometimes too thin, while anyone with a slow metabolic rate tends to store some foods in the form of surplus fat.

We must have protein every day because the body cannot store it. Protein is a must in any diet, for it helps to replace the worn-out cells and tissues of the body.

So never cut down on meat, fish, cheese, eggs and milk. They do not put on weight if you keep to your one cooked meal a day.

A certain amount of fats, sugars and starches are essential for fuel and energy, but the body can store these, so we can afford to cut down on them.

It is essential, however, to eat what is really good for us and most of us need bread. I personally prefer brown bread, which I still think is best, although I am told that full vitamins are put into white bread for those who prefer it. Opinions vary on the fattening qualities of potatoes. I have them several times a week – boiled with a knob of butter but never with bread at the same meal. *Puddings and cakes, much as I love them, I will not eat.* I like fresh fruit for a sweet, or of course cheese. I ignore the biscuits and jam, but honey is excellent – a real pick-me-up when feeling low and when tension builds and tummies suffer, it is easily digested.

The whole thing is really a question of not being able to have your cake and eat it too. If there is a food you particularly like and it does you good and is difficult to give up, well, give up something else to balance your intake, so that you can have it. But don't try to build your youth and beauty on starches, fats and sugars; you must have protein, vegetables, fruit and salads to a much greater degree. These foods will put the shine into you, the vitality, the youthfulness, the staying power and the ability to do the things you have to do and want to do.

If you are a wonderful cook, it must be very difficult to refuse the gorgeous confections you make for your family, but to some extent feeding the family and visitors is getting simpler. So many people of all ages are becoming figure conscious that they would almost welcome a slimming meal, providing there is plenty of variety.

When putting on weight, which I do all too easily, I wage a cold war on my appetite by eating cold food. This gets my weight down a little faster, which is sometimes necessary if I am to take a Keep Fit Rally or make a special personal appearance.

One of the pitfalls to avoid is a nice cup of coffee and a snack. It is friendly and sociable, I agree, but eating between meals never was any good for the figure. Neither, I think, is drinking with meals. Far better always to leave the tea or coffee to last.

Picnic meals can be difficult. Not the fun ones, because there is usually time to get them organized, but the daily 'sandwich to work'. If necessary, I take the kind of food I eat normally – brown bread, salad, egg, cheese, cold lean meat, and fruit, but I never touch that lovely bar of chocolate that can be so tempting for afterwards. I try to buy fruit and not sweets.

How I love the salads in the spring! The first tiny spring onions, the radishes, the endive, the watercress, and the chicory – the beauty foods. I believe in olive oil as a beauty treatment, inside and out, so I have this or lemon juice as a dressing and the only time I ever touch white sugar is when I have a little on my lettuce – I always prefer brown for sweetening.

Many women who may have to attend business lunches or banquets with their husbands say that keeping to a diet is difficult in these circumstances. 'Besides,' I am often told, 'it's not polite to pick and choose and refuse courses, especially if you are being entertained in a private home.' I think that having dinner in a private house is the only occasion on which I would ignore a diet completely and pay my hostess the courtesy of eating what is set in front of me. I could make up for it the next day by cutting out all bread and potatoes!

However, it is perfectly easy to order sensibly from a menu at a business lunch or to skip certain courses on a public banquet menu without offending anyone.

When having a meal in a restaurant I might choose from the menu as follows: Melon or shrimp cocktail rather than hors d'oeuvres, soup or pâté. Plain fish, chicken or meat with salad or a green vegetable rather than made-up dishes like curry or the chef's special. I never order potatoes with the main course, but prefer a second green vegetable. For a third course I like cheese to eat with one piece of crisp bread or a fruit salad with a little cream. Coffee to follow. I never eat a roll and butter with my meal, and prefer not to drink with it – although a small glass of red Burgundy wine is hard to resist with a good steak and is a very good pick-me-up!

The Keep Fit way of eating is not cheap, but then neither are the cakes, sweets, and pastries which often push up the housekeeping budget. Better food and less of it is my watchword. It seems so silly to me to overwork the digestive organs by giving them a lot of unnecessary fillers which do us no real good. As we accustom ourselves to eating in this new way, our stomachs very obligingly adjust themselves to the lower intake.

Over-eating is ageing because it causes overweight, breathlessness and heavy, laboured movement. Stay young by eating sensibly, shunning too many starchy and fat foods and eating all the wonderful foods that are so good for you – vegetables, fruit, cheese, butter, all the fish in the sea, meat, eggs and milk. These are the glamour foods, high in precious vitamins that will give you health, vitality and youth.

Perhaps you'd like to know my simple daily routine.

I've got a funny little tea-pot which was given to me years ago. It's very small and I always make my early morning tea in this. I make it very weak and I drink it immediately – otherwise it gives me indigestion.

**Breakfast**

The juice of two or three oranges, one piece of toast and butter and an apple is plenty in the summer, but in the winter a boiled egg or small plate of porridge or cereal keeps me warm. Anyone facing a long journey to work might need bacon and eggs or scrambled egg and tomato, but never endless fattening pieces of toast and butter.

**Mid morning**

If I need a weak coffee, I have it – or it could be tea or Bovril. But this is only if I'm exercising hard. I don't need it if I'm writing.

**Lunch**

Usually light – ham or egg salad, or cheese and cracker biscuits, followed by fruit (but not bananas).

**Dinner**

Casserole of fresh meat and vegetables or lamb chop, or occasionally poultry. Boiled potatoes some days, or brown bread, and mostly green vegetables. For a sweet I eat fresh fruit or stewed fruit, cheese, or an egg custard.

And I have reasonable helpings of everything – as I said before, I still love to eat.

# 4 Relaxation

For many of us life is like a treadmill. We are afraid to stop, afraid to relax in case we cannot get going again. What a terrible mistake we are making! Unless we relax we cannot stop on the treadmill.

For some of us it is easy to relax but others have lost the art of letting go. We must learn to drift sometimes with the tide, to go with it and not against it. Relaxation is almost more important than the ability to sleep. Not everyone is lost to the world in sleep; some toss and turn and even talk while the subconscious mind refuses to let them go, and they wake unrefreshed.

These days it is more important than ever to learn the art of relaxation, to shut out at times the man-made turmoil and slip into a state of stillness and peace. How to do it?

Well, first things first. Do you know when you are tense? Or do you wait until the back of your neck feels knotted up, your back aches, so does your head, and you feel slightly sick? Never get to that stage. Put yourself into a state of tension now. Imagine something frightful is happening. Screw yourself up in a panic of nerves, then suddenly, blissfully, let go. Stretch out your arm and hold it rigid, every muscle and nerve straining to keep it there. Then drop it so that it flops heavily and limply into your lap. In other words, relax it. Every time you feel that tightening of the skin, muscles and nerves, let go, because tension can kill. Utter fatigue through nervous exhaustion poisons the system and leaves you grey and old. Refresh yourself mentally and physically by learning to let go.

Keep Fit taught me to do this. I was the world's worst worrier. If I had nothing to worry about, that worried me too. I just didn't realize what was happening to me. How I exhausted myself! I know now. I learnt to relax through muscular relaxation and moving to music. It has been a great blessing.

I had always danced and I loved it; I started to learn my first steps at three years old. But this was not the same thing at all – this curious therapy of happiness that we call 'Keep Fit'. Stretching and relaxing, always relaxing, not struggling to reach examination standard or to stay up on our toes, just moving to the best of our ability, but somehow always moving on.

For obvious reasons the exercise did me good physically – but there was more to it than that. How quickly my fatigue disappeared and I felt refreshed again, relaxed in body and mind!

As I sit in my studio writing this I can see my neighbour's washing on the line. It's Monday morning and a lovely day. I do hope she won't be too tired to enjoy it. Why do so many of us feel it necessary to exhaust ourselves because it is Monday? Spread the work and remember that lovely days are rare enough to be treasured because they are good for you as well as for your washing.

Relax . . . relax . . . Have you ever tried rubbing the back of your neck very gently for a few minutes? It never fails to make me sleepy – in fact I nearly always yawn. Tension often shows in the hands before anywhere else and it helps to relieve this if you close and open them strongly, shake them and let them flop in your lap.

One young woman wrote to me telling me of her joy in recovering the use of her hands after a year of being unable to move them. She had been giving piano lessons at a school for some years when she suddenly began to lose the mobility of her fingers. There seemed to be no valid physical reason and neither she nor her doctor could discover why or how it had come about. Gradually her finger movements became almost completely inhibited and she lost her job and went home to her parents.

One afternoon she was looking in at TV when I happened to be demonstrating some hand exercises. These are among my favourite exercises and I practice them often, for my hands are not my pride and joy (although they might be called the joy of the gipsies, so lined and creased are they that they must have a long story to tell, and nothing gives me greater pleasure than to be told that they look graceful in movement).

The young teacher watched and was infuriated when I happened to remark casually that, 'anyone can do these exercises'. She had the set switched off and confessed later that she had felt like throwing something at it. But a moment later she could not resist having another peek and the set was switched on again. She began to try and copy the hand movements and afterwards practised them daily, struggling to regain the use of her fingers. A year later she wrote to tell me that she was now back in her teaching post and regarded her recovery as a miracle. To me it is just added proof that physical exercises can and do have a remedial effect on nervous troubles, provided there is the will to do them.

Mind and body are so linked that deliberate physical relaxation cannot fail to have its effect on our nerves and minds.

My TV team of housewives know this only too well. Often when we rehearsed for the programme I was overcome by a feeling of remorse at working my faithful band so hard all morning.

'Come on,' I would say, 'we'll do some relaxing exercises.'

Helen, my accompanist, would begin to play 'Lazybones' and I would lower my voice to a murmur. Then we would start stretching and relaxing exercises on the floor and the team were soon lulled into such an advanced state of sleepiness that it took all my persuasive powers to make them get up off the floor! 'For goodness sake, Eileen,' they would implore, 'don't put that in the programme.' It appalled them to imagine what millions of television viewers would think if they were to see Eileen Fowler's lively Keep Fit team going to sleep before their very eyes.

The exercises on pages 82–84 are those that we use for relaxing.

Finally, it is easy to relax when the sun is shining and all is well; but when we are worried and live in fear, it's not so easy. There is only one way to relax mind and body completely all the time – it is to have faith, to face up to a problem and say to yourself, 'I will work, I will struggle but I will not fret, for an answer will surely be found.'

# 5 Sleep

My fifth and final Golden Key to staying young is Sleep – sound, refreshing sleep. I suppose we can have too much but I doubt whether this applies to the average woman. Her problem is to get enough, enough to keep her looking fresh, to keep her face unlined, to make her glad to get up in the morning and able to cope with whatever lies before her. These essentials form the only yardstick by which she can really measure the amount she needs. Individual requirements vary so much. One usually reads that eight hours is enough when we are young and that the older we get the less we need.

This I find hard to believe. If you can lead a regular life it may work, but how many of us can do this? Today a woman leads the kind of life into which she must fit her sleeping hours as best she can; glamour jobs, shift work, teenagers living at home, television, or illness all tend to disrupt her design for living and she is lucky if she can get off to sleep at the same time for several nights in succession. I do not think this matters as long as she gets all the sleep she needs. I still think that an hour before midnight is worth two after, but this is not everyone's opinion.

If you can go to bed at any time and automatically fall asleep to wake a few hours later, bright faced and dewy eyed, I should skip what follows and be thankful; but if, like me, you cannot do this, well, see if my personal experience will help you.

The long run of weekly television programmes convinced me that I had to take a more realistic attitude to sleep. Creative work, teaching, hours of travelling and rehearsal made facing the cameras a bit of a hazard. Not only must I do the job, but I must always look the part. A singer could have a relaxed throat, a dancer a sprained ankle, but Eileen Fowler says, 'Do what I say and it will keep you fit.' How could I be ill, or look desperately tired? I couldn't explain to viewers that I was under strain and needed a rest from my own words of wisdom!

I realized that sleep was the answer. So somehow I got it. I learnt never to go past the point of no return; never to say, 'I must finish this tonight if it kills me.' I went to bed early and got up and did my work in the early morning. I learnt to sleep in the train – an undreamed of talent – and every hour's sleep I lost, I made up somehow. I have done it ever since. I force the problem out of my mind and stop. If I don't, I cannot bear to look in the mirror and I am tired and irritable.

Work when you must, for just as long as you must, and then stop or you will make those tired lines round your eyes permanent and that droop to your mouth will never go. How can it be otherwise? You are training your face that way by being too tired to smile and lift the corners of your mouth, too tired to keep a happy, relaxed expression that will keep you young-looking and pretty.

Sleep is the best beauty treatment of all. While we sleep, there is a renewal within us, both mental and physical.

Supposing when you get to bed you cannot sleep. Sleeping pills are seldom the right answer. In cases of chronic insomnia and under doctor's orders they may help, but the demand for sleeping drug prescriptions has reached frightening proportions in this country.

It is far better to cultivate sleep as a good habit – slowly but surely. It helps me to sleep if I open windows wide and draw curtains back. I never sleep on a soft bed and although I don't like too many bedclothes, I must be warm; my circulation is not my strong point when I am immobile so I like a bottle or electric blanket. To prevent a double chin I have as low a pillow as I can bear.

Late meals do not help, so it's better not to eat anything heavy after 7.30 in the evening. Indigestion is one of the causes of insomnia. Constipation and flatulence are enemies of sleep. If the cause is emotional, sleep only comes as a result of sheer exhaustion.

If you have time to relax before you go to bed, that's fine, but if not, practise your stretching and relaxing in bed, then try to think of yourself as being made of lead. Muscles, once relaxed, mercifully go on relaxing. So start with your feet; imagine that they are so heavy you can't lift them; then your knees, hips, shoulders and head. Try to lift your head off the pillow, but feel that you cannot – it's too heavy. Then try to empty your mind, and imagine that you are floating on a beautiful lake.

If you do all this and find it is still a lot of no good, take time off next day to discover the real cause for your sleeplessness. Far better to face up to something that is worrying you than to try to ignore it, because it is there, rooted in your subconscious mind and will go on nagging and keeping you awake. If there is a problem that is keeping you awake at night, get advice from someone you can trust and do something about it straight away. Dig it out and get rid of it. Don't live with fear and worry if you can possibly help it, because they won't let you sleep – and sleep will keep you young.

# 6 The young ones

If you want to be full of life, with the sort of casual elegance that draws all eyes and is right for every occasion, well, why not? You can, if you work at it. Keep Fit will keep you the way you want to be.

When I look around me at the teenage girls of today I am struck by their potential beauty. Yet most of the younger girls I meet seem to be over-critical of their own shortcomings. They worry about their faces and figures. Their standard is high and they cannot imagine that the years will correct their puppy fat or their few figure faults.

So how can one tell the teenage girl that nothing is more detrimental to an attractive appearance than self-consciousness, that it only serves to draw attention to the failings that concern her most? Of course, she longs to be what she considers beautiful at the moment. What girl worth her salt doesn't? Here is an age of discovery, when she develops that weapon which keeps every woman on her toes and anxious to stay attractive all her life – feminine vanity.

There is a bridge to be crossed between childhood and womanhood and many a teenager nowadays is over-anxious to cross it quickly. It is a fact that Keep Fit will help her to cross that bridge gracefully. I have seen it work. From 1934 to 1945 I had Industrial Keep Fit Classes in so many factories that eventually it became necessary to have other Leaders on my staff. The classes I took personally included one of girls from nine to fifteen, the children of my grown-up members. It was an unusual group for Keep

Fit because girls of this age receive their physical education at school and normally require nothing further.

My assistant and I adored these young terrors. They were as keen as mustard and couldn't get enough dancing or movement training, throwing themselves into it with wonderful enthusiasm, yet the task of keeping sixty girls of that age in order was more than exhausting. They were not badly behaved; they were simply so full of life that discipline was a farce. However, we won in the end and a livelier and lovelier clutch of teenagers we could not have wished to see.

Those six years of training in poise, charm and movement resulted in confident, pleasing personalities and slim, supple and rounded figures. Within a year or two all were married and having babies; today they are back in an afternoon class run by one of my old students, now a gracious and experienced leader.

The right kind of exercise will do something for a girl who is learning to be a woman. We have all seen the girl who turns heads everywhere she goes. She may not be strictly beautiful, but there is something indefinable about her. Personality? Poise? Vitality? Yes, perhaps, yet there is something more. She is walking beautifully, as if the world belongs to her – head up, shoulders down, spine erect – and because of this, she looks beautiful.

Anyone can join a Keep Fit Class at fifteen and because of the increasing interest shown by the younger age-groups I have for some time been working on a 'top twenty' approach.

Dancing the modern way is a good beginning to beauty for any girl, but if that girl wants to go one step farther and fashion her growing figure so that her clothes fit beautifully, so that she can enter a room full of strangers with confidence and poise, so that she walks and moves gracefully all her life, then she should learn to stretch and bend and twist and swing to her favourite music.

Many youth clubs have classes where a modern mixture of dancing and Keep Fit is very popular.

The early marriage age of today sometimes means that a girl will give up her classes at nineteen or twenty, but it is my experience that she always comes back to them a year or two later – once a Keep Fit girl, always a Keep Fit girl!

Have you yourself any young figure problems? If so, turn to page 89. These Teenage exercises will give you some slimming movements for the waistline, tummy and hips. There is also a push-up movement for the bust-line.

If this type of Keep Fit is new to you, I would certainly start at the beginning with standing, sitting and walking tall. Follow the instructions and you will look and feel more attractive at once. You are used to the latest dances so that bending your knees will be a 'natural'; but take the trouble to learn the basic movements properly so that the exercises really do something for your poise and figure.

With your enormous variety of pop and classical records you are bound to find some tempos that will fit the movements. Your transistor will help, too. Don't rush the movements. Remember that your muscles need training to hold you in shape as you mature.

'Sensible Eating' will also help you to fine down your figure and give you a plan to work on, but don't forget that you are still growing and developing, so don't cut down on food too suddenly, thinking that it will help, because it won't.

Gradually ease off the schoolgirl meals and begin to pick and choose a bit, watching that what you are eating is nourishing and not just plain stodge. Don't miss a meal. It won't help to go without food for hours at a time; even a youngster can look drawn and tired without regular meals and enough rest. You are bound to lose some sleep while you are out enjoying yourself, but make it up, or your looks and vitality will suffer – so will everybody else's in the family!

If you want to add inches, you should still exercise, but more slowly, and try to think about the muscles you are using at the time. I have always found that thin girls benefit just as much from exercise as those with curves; they find it relaxing – which is half the battle in their attempt to put on weight.

Many girls and women tell me that they would like to increase the bust-line measurement. This is not easy because the bust itself is mostly glandular, and any attempt to enlarge it usually means putting on weight everywhere else as well. However, exercise will improve your appearance by developing the chest muscles, so that the breasts have a natural lift. Deeper breathing, the 'good posture' training, soon make a big difference to the way your dress sits at the front. It is the constant lift which goes right through these exercises which does it.

The teenager on page 92 is picking up a book weighing about 1½lb (680gm) and is circling it slowly up and round. The extra weight makes the uplift muscles work a little harder and therefore they become more toned up and more developed. I was a late developer in my teens and literally fashioned my neck, chest and shoulders with exercise. I did it to get into proportion with my hips, which were fairly wide. I swam a lot too, which helped. See 'Sit and Swim' on page 79.

If you are very small in the bust, a 32-in. bra with an 'A' cup is somewhere to start. Shop around until you find one that really fits you. Get advice from an expert – many big stores have them on their staff.

While you are developing your chest, don't be shy about wearing a bra that is slightly built up. It will restore your confidence and you are less likely to droop, which many slim girls do – particularly the tall ones – thinking that this makes their flat chest less noticeable. If you are tall, be proud of your height. Many of us would give a great deal to have those extra inches.

Check the way you stand regularly. If only by lining up, back against a wall – not stiffly but relaxing on to it so that your back touches most of the way down. Walk away in that position. It may seem wrong, but it's right.

It is important to remember that a small bust, to look as full as possible, needs a slim waistline and a very flat tummy. Never slump or let your back go; tummy muscles work with back muscles and they will slacken too.

Have you tried ten-pin bowling? I did and discovered that it's good fun and a real figure-trimmer. Like everyone else, I had beginner's luck at first and found that my Keep Fit training helped me considerably. Bending the knees, keeping in the tummy and seat, as you roll the ball down the alley has much the same effect as some of our Keep Fit exercises. Relaxation is very important, too, for a winning style – watch the experts and the ease with which they play.

Bowling can keep you slim and supple when short evenings and bad weather make other outdoor forms of exercise impossible.

So can Keep Fit, of course, and you can use it as a base for other skills. Why not try it?

# 7 Stay the girl he married

When I see a young woman out shopping, sometimes accompanied by small children, always with an abstracted look in her eye as she calculates the family budget, I often find myself counting off on my fingers the different people that she must be – wife, mother, housekeeper, playmate and wise counsellor – the list is endless. But I often pause to wonder, too, how she is managing her life and the many rôles that she has to play. Perhaps it is you I am looking at. What will you do today? Will you work hard and still have time to play? Will you bring a sense of enjoyment to everything that you do?

Will you stay the girl he married?

If you are in your twenties or early thirties it is probable that you will finish the day healthily tired and able to pick up energy again very quickly. But what will happen when you reach your forties? Will you still find enjoyment in life, finishing the day feeling fit and looking fit, with a glorious sense of achievement at work well done? The answer to that question depends on how you live today.

Now is the time to build. Now, when you are building your family, your fortunes, your friends, build health for the future by the way that you spend each day. Say to yourself: 'I will stay young because I want always to get the maximum enjoyment from life.'

The Five Golden Keys to staying young are very important to anyone who is looking ahead to years of health and beauty. But it is often the housewife, the woman one would think has the freedom to arrange her own day so that she lives wisely, who squanders all her energy on the demands of her household.

Any young wife, if she really tries, can fit the rules of health into her busy life. Ten minutes a day spent doing special exercises will keep her fit and supple. I usually do my exercises in the morning in between the odd chores. This is convenient because then I have my comfortable clothes on.

Attending a Keep Fit Class once a week is a wonderful way of keeping an interest that will take a woman outside the home. More than a million women in Britain today belong to various Keep Fit and health organizations, not counting those who exercise daily in their homes. There is a strong social side for anyone who is a newcomer to a town or country district. If there is no Keep Fit Class near you, why not start one yourself? The information on page 14 will tell you how to go about it.

**Working wives**

If you have a job and a home to run as well you will have very little time to yourself. I am well aware that a job often keeps a woman mentally young, lively, interesting and more capable of being an attractive and intelligent companion to her husband. This is particularly true of a woman who is working because she wants to. If, however, a wife leaves her home for hours at a time because, for some reason or other, it is absolutely necessary, it can take a great toll on her physical health.

This must be watched very carefully and I would strongly advise you to follow our Five Golden Keys; the more mental and physical energy you pour out, the more you need their help. The human battery needs recharging from time to time to give constant service, and time must be found to fulfil these needs. With so much to do, it is vital to use any spare minutes to catch up on your energy. Nervous exhaustion is your enemy, so keep it at bay by relaxing whenever you can.

If you have a meal to get immediately on your return from work and you are dead on your feet, slip off your shoes and do the upside-down exercise. You will see it on page 83. It will work wonders! Lie flat on the floor with feet up on the end of a bed or, if you are alone, on the chair in the kitchen, while the oven is warming up or the kettle is boiling. Until you've tried it you cannot imagine how it feels to have your feet higher than your head and the blood flowing into your face. It releases the tensions of the day and any weary or drawn look fades away and leaves you fresh and rested for the evening. Try it!

**Housewives**

In contrast to the working wives, the stay-at-home mother of small children often feels shut-in. A day spent indoors with children who may be off-colour and fractious can be terribly wearing. Trying to keep the children happy and at the same time get through one hundred and one niggling jobs can suddenly make you want to push the walls away and get out.

Well, push them away. Go on! Let's stand in the middle of the room with feet apart and that wretched brush in one hand. Let's swing it up and round in circles, rocking and swinging and stretching until we are moving with such freedom that we've all the space we need. Even if it's 'pouring cats and dogs,' let's open the windows to the wide world and take some deep breaths. Let's get the children to join in. It's fun. It's even more fun to music. A favourite record or Radio Two and we're off. Soon the blissful easing of tension can be recognized and we feel human once more.

There are so many ways in which housewives can save themselves and learn to relax. Believe me, it's all too easy to forget this. We hunch shoulders and battle our way through the day, buzzing from one task to the next with speed but little grace, and finishing the day a wreck.

Let's think how we can improve things. Are we firm with ourselves? Do we do so much housework in a day and no more? That takes as much discipline for some of us as it does for others to be houseproud. Can you sit with your feet up for a moment while the housework waits, untroubled by that nagging guilt complex so many of us suffer from? If you can then you're my kind of girl. We can learn to get ahead with our chores during the time we feel energetic. The table that needs polishing, the doorstep that needs cleaning, how important are they? They will be here when we're dead!

I am a bit houseproud myself but I fight it. I refuse to let the house run me. I try to save myself all the time. I keep a low stool under the kitchen table and kick it out and put my feet on it at the slightest opportunity. Any jobs that can be done sitting, I do, and if there's a patch of sunlight from an open window, my chair goes there. I hate being indoors so I take all possible jobs into the garden and do them there. My summer tan is pure Thames Estuary, but it looks much the same as the South of France variety.

Housework is a necessary evil, but I don't see why it should take toll of our looks. I am full of admiration for the woman who spring-cleans and still manages to look pretty while she is doing it.

Thank goodness more and more slacks are worn in the home. It's so much safer when clambering up steps or moving heavy furniture. Many accidents in the home are caused by attempting some gymnastic feat for which neither the clothes nor muscles are prepared.

**After-baby figures**

Modern mothers expect to regain their vitality and their figures after childbirth, and fifty per cent of my letters from viewers and listeners are requests for information on this subject. As every case is individual and requires specialized advice, I always reply in this way:

Most young mothers return to Keep Fit Classes from three to six months after their baby is born and always with their doctor's permission. Some mothers are very strong and can begin to exercise like this as soon as they finish feeding the baby but others need longer to recover enough strength and stamina to join in a fairly vigorous class. The stretching and relaxing method of moving is infinitely suitable for new mothers, providing a start is not made too soon.

If you are beginning to move to music at home, start gently, first making sure that you have medical permission to do so. The first basic movements are what you need. Standing tall, relaxing, rocking from foot to foot, bending your knees, easy stretching and swinging and simple tummy exercises on the floor. Hip exercises are good too. Limber up gently and you will find you will move more and more until you regain your slim figure and your vitality.

Make use of the Five Golden Keys – the keys are fashioned for you. Exercise, fresh air, sensible eating, relaxation, and sleep. Use them to stay young, and the girl he married.

# 8 The gracious years

Why are we so age-conscious, I wonder? Is it because we think in terms of those wretched 'three-score years and ten'; because legally our age is limited for us? Old age for women at sixty, for instance?

I shall never forget the shock I got when a member of my Television Keep Fit Team said one day, 'In a few years' time, Eileen, you'll be able to ride on the Birmingham trams for nothing!' I am all for a bit of help as I get older, but I believe in thinking young. What would have happened if Sir Winston Churchill had thought that he was too old at sixty-five to lead us through a World War? I know that retirement is necessary to give the young ones a chance, but why shouldn't we make it a starting point for something else? Another vital interest to keep us young for ever.

Think young – feel young. . . . Of one thing I am certain, get through middle-age and you are away – a second spring if you like. Get your second wind and on you go, and what fun it is when you know some of the answers! Mind you, I didn't always think like this.

One summer evening a long time ago my first attack of giddiness resulted in a fall from the top of the grand piano. I was taking a Keep Fit Class in an overcrowded gymnasium and I had got up on the piano so that those at the back could see my feet. That's about all they did see for some minutes. Everyone said that it was the heat so I promptly forgot all about it. That was the first time. There were others.

Finally I went to my doctor – a specialist in women's

ailments. 'You need a hysterectomy,' he said, and operated immediately. He explained carefully that this would be an enforced change – unnatural but necessary.

Apparently some women cross the menopause bridge with serenity and health, wondering what all the fuss is about. Others need an operation as I did. Some sail through naturally; others, highly strung and imaginative, find it affects the nervous system to a greater or lesser degree. I learnt, however, much to my relief, that any problems would be physical, and not mental, and all part of the glandular changes that go on at this time. It was quite unnecessary to battle through on my own when medical help was at hand.

I took my prescription thankfully and went back to my teaching. Of course, I overdid it and made no attempt to adjust my life in any way. I had been told to rest as much as possible, to relax, and that any wage-earning woman should remember that it is her health which allows her to earn, so she should allot a percentage of those years to a real holiday – and a restful one. It all sounded so 'old' to me, so I took no notice.

Before long I had to. One day I was young and vital, the next middle-aged, bored and depressed. My doctor patiently repeated the reasons for my misery. I realized that I must help myself.

That Christmas, a friend gave me an American beauty book. Reading it shook me to the core. I knew that I already had most of the know-how, but was failing to apply it to myself.

From that moment I was a changed woman. I told myself that in five years I would be fifty so I began to plan for the time when life would begin again in a different kind of way. First to reduce my weight, to lose 1½ stone (9.5kg.); to get rid of sluggishness, indigestion and headaches; to guard against colds and back-ache. I resolved to look after my hair, eyes and teeth; to change some of my ideas about clothes and make-up; to shop locally for my pretties – I was too nervous to board a train.

This was when I began to realize the value of sleep and real relaxation. Bit by bit I fought back with the Five Golden Keys I have told you about, and blissfully they worked.

Within three years I was on television! I was forty-eight and not exactly a Cleopatra, but they were looking for a Keep Fit instructress – not too young and not too old – so they chose me. That was twenty years ago.

Now I know that any woman can stay young and start a new career if she wants to at any age. We have the power within ourselves to do so, providing we want to enough and are willing to work towards this end.

If you have days when you feel that you are not living but merely existing, then do something about it.

Start with a medical check-up – you must have the right base to work on.

Look at yourself in a long mirror.

What will you change? Everything? Certainly not. Your neck, bust-line, legs and ankles may be excellent, but perhaps you could slim your waistline, hips and thighs, flatten tummy and seat. And what about your shoulders? Have you let them round a little, so that a pad of fat is sitting at the top of your back? That could become a dowager's hump if neglected. Upper arms – are they flabby? Do your feet ache at times? Then find the answer to all these problems with the Five Golden Keys.

You needn't be afraid to do the exercises, but start gently. Get limbered up and, if possible, join a Keep Fit Class. Make a point of stretching upwards every day to pull your bust away from your hips. Do the floor exercises frequently to strengthen tummy and back muscles. Bend and swing and dance around. You are not too old at any age for this, but if for any good reason you find sitting a *must*, then there are mobility exercises for you to do in a chair. Your watchwords are Exercise and Sensible Eating. Never forget them if you want to stay slim.

Think again about clothes. Top sophistication can be so attractive in the thirties and early forties, but I found that it helped me to look younger if I avoided too much obvious glamour in the fifties. No over-tight suits, frilly blouses, very high heels or comic hats. I prefer a jersey suit or dress, beautifully tailored, a straight coat or Burberry, soft beret exactly to tone, and beautiful shoes, stockings and gloves. You can look like a girl in clothes like these, if you have good posture, vitality and a happy smile.

Many English women carry most of their weight below the waistline and often feel that they must wear a full skirt to disguise it. Add a fitted top and the whole effect is pear-shaped. A straight skirt with pleat at the back for freedom and a looser, longer top changes the whole line and puts it into proportion. (See Exercises for tummy and thigh.)

Have fewer clothes in your wardrobe, but let them be of beautiful materials, texture and colour, and tailored by someone who knows his job. 'Classic' clothes need not be 'mannish'. Well lined jersey suits in off-beat colours can be most feminine and becoming.

Unless you are tall and slender, work for a longer effect from head to toe. Avoid anything that makes you look shorter and broader. If your shoulders are wide, leave high necked, light tops alone (dark ones with 'V' necks are kinder) and cover the tops of your arms. Most of the year I find that dark, plain materials help me to look taller and slimmer but, if I have to wear one, I like a light hat. I have a weakness for very plain 'creamy-to-coffee'-coloured gloves – the type that wrinkle elegantly around the wrist – fabric usually and very washable. I always have a spare pair in my brief-case when I go to Town.

Foundation garments are often a problem and usually require an expert's advice. For some figures an overall support is necessary but they give me a solid, one-piece feeling and seem to drag the bust-line down towards the hips – the very thing we are trying to avoid. I would suggest sensible eating and exercise to reduce a roll around the waistline, a really good belt – not too long – and an uplift bra. The midriff is then mobile and will give an impression of suppleness and youth.

**Head to toe beauty**

Having made daily exercise and sensible eating a regular habit, relaxation, more sleep and fresh air part of your daily life, let's gild the lily.

How about your hair? Go for natural, healthy hair with a modern line. Don't be persuaded to try out all the latest dyes and bleaches unless your hairdresser is very, very experienced.

Hair can look lovely these days if you insist on putting its fitness first. Don't over-bleach like I did once. It took a very long time to get my hair right again. Now I watch its condition. Every morning I loosen the scalp by moving it around with the tips of my fingers; a tight scalp is one of the greatest enemies of healthy hair. For extreme dryness I like an olive-oil soaking before a shampoo.

As a general rule short hair is youthful, a long bob practically never, past teenage. Too much 'teased-out width' tends to broaden the silhouette. Here again we need line – a good headline. If facial bone structure is good, close cropping can give elegance at ninety.

I think a modern hairstyle is very important – not, of course, one so extreme that it hardens the features, but the right cutting and shaping which softens facial contours and is right up to date.

Faces are to some extent what we make them. Curious little mannerisms tend to creep in quite unnoticed by ourselves. Pursing of the lips causes little vertical lines; tension and raised foreheads, horizontal ones; unhappy thoughts cause a drooping of the whole face, the corners of the mouth in particular.

Don't let this happen to you! Be on the watch and relax your face, even if you've nothing to smile about. Know when you are tense and let go. I am doing this now. I have just seen my own grim look in the mirror, and although I am really enjoying every minute, concentration can be ugly. Watch its effects and counteract them.

Take care of your eyes, too. Peering at something you can no longer see easily, can be very ageing. Strained eyes tend to sink into your head and look smaller. If glasses are a *must*, try a prescription for some dark ones for summer, and choose really attractive frames for general use.

If you've still kept all your own teeth you probably feel rather smug and young, and of course modern cosmetic dentistry can take years off your appearance, if the teeth are rather worn-looking. Twenty-volume peroxide can help to keep them sparkling and the gums firm. Soak a tiny pad of cotton wool in peroxide and dab it on, but use both hands alternately to do this because it is rather drying for the fingertips. I do this about once a week in addition to brushing my teeth as often as possible.

I realize now that for years I used too much make-up; an allergy which caused eyelids and lips to swell and irritate put an end to that. I was forced to go to a skin specialist who advised cleansing with olive oil, then a little lacto-calamine and no soap and water. A glowing non-allergic lipstick kept me happy and also provided a little colour, high on my cheeks. My skin has never looked back. I like a little good powder – warm in tone. I make up my eyelashes on occasions but seldom use eye-shadow. I have lost a somewhat dingy look which came from clogged pores, and am not constantly employed 'renewing my face'. Now my pennies go on perfume instead.

However, I do wash my neck with soap and water! and it gets preferential treatment in every way. This is a real danger zone and must be kept youthful.

If face and neck are inclined to be dry and line easily, cleanse both with olive oil at bedtime and massage and slap lightly with a nourishing skin food. Remove surplus cream and splash with cold water in the morning, bathing your eyes at the same time. If you dislike any semblance of a tan, a cut lemon keeps the skin white and gives a fresher look to the face. If the skin reddens, coat with lacto-calamine.

Good posture will do the rest, and that means practising the exercises for a double chin, neck and shoulders – page 75.

My hands need extra care and I give it to them. I wear gloves for house jobs and keep a good hand-cream or jelly by my bed and sink, and a cut lemon too for stains. A pinky-brown polish suits my nails best, and here again, with smaller make-up costs, I can buy a really good one. If you have beautiful hands, then you can go to Town and highlight them, attracting all the attention you can get, but whatever their attributes, use them beautifully. Relax them, because tension often shows first in the hands and results in fidgety, jarring, ugly little movements. Let them speak for you, but they must speak well. See Fascinating Fingers, page 80.

**Happy feet**

'You are as old as your feet.' So spake the oracle – my French grandmother. Such pretty little feet she had, and so strong. She exercised them, put them up whenever she could and bought them very good shoes. My mother could wear them – they were too small for me. 'My feet must be happy,' she would say, 'and they will take me anywhere.' She made her dresses and hats exquisitely and spent the money she saved on her shoes. I am no needlewoman unfortunately, but good shoes I will have, if I go without something else in order to buy them.

Elegance and comfort cost money – spend that money on your shoes. It will save your face, your figure, your energy and your youth.

# 9 Keeping fit

Why not join your local Keep Fit Class or start one yourself? If you have moved to a new town or a modern block of flats you may be missing the fun you had with old friends and neighbours. Well, you can get a similar kind of fun at a Keep Fit Class. You laugh a lot, and it's all very friendly.

No one worries if a newcomer gets a bit tangled up the first time. The others giggle with you, remembering their own short-comings when they started themselves. Very soon everyone is swinging and stretching in unison.

The music helps, of course, as much of it is familiar. You cannot help relaxing and when it is time to go home, you are all toned-up and mentally refreshed.

Then, of course, there is the Leader who wins the confidence of her class members by doing her dedicated best to turn them into a set of glamorous sylphs. Before long she has you moving to music for your figure, and the sheer love of it.

Last, but never least, there is the pianist. One minute she has your toes twinkling to her irresistible rhythm – the next you are elegant and poised as you move to her improvised melodies. She is with you from the first note, and never too tired to take that movement just once again.

Keep Fit demonstrations are popular because it is fun to improve your own performance sufficiently to take part and on the day to make members of the audience want to join a class themselves.

During the war in Essex, Middlesex and Hertfordshire Keep Fit Pageants given by my Industrial Group were regular events – hundreds of girls and women taking part. Specially picked teams of Leaders, their slim, tanned figures dressed in white, were a joy to see and they declare now that they owe their present-day health and vitality to those open-air activities.

Nowadays displays of all kinds are run by Keep Fit organizations all over the country. Thousands watch the pageantry of movement and colour which overnight turns an audience into Keep Fit fans.

The rallies, too, are tremendous fun. Halls are booked a year ahead. Fast, modern, streamlined coaches from places miles apart disgorge their eager load. Excitement runs high, and the chatter too, but when the Leader appears and the music starts, the chatter dies away and there is only room for rhythm and a joy of moving to music. At tea-time, strangers no longer, the members get together and chatter again. What about? Keep Fit, I guess!

I hope I shall meet you at a rally some day. Good-bye!

# Exercises

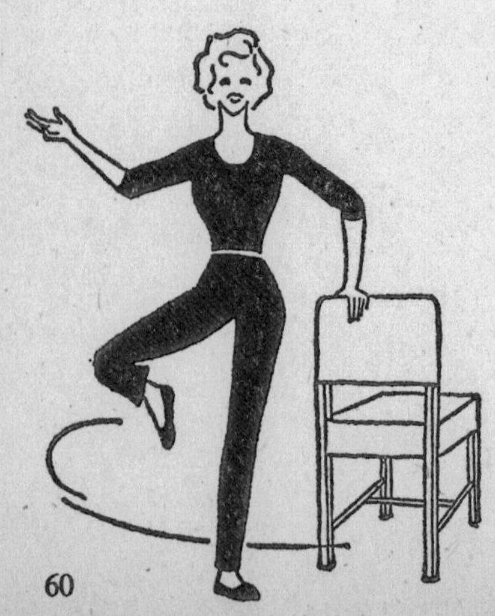

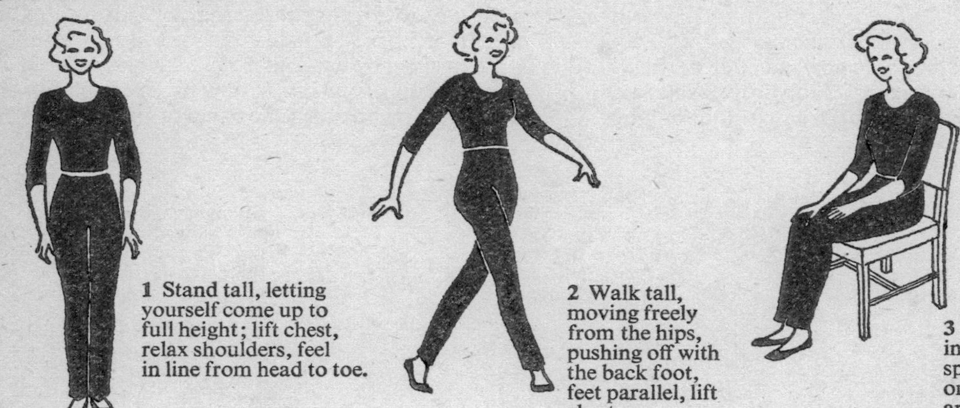

1 Stand tall, letting yourself come up to full height; lift chest, relax shoulders, feel in line from head to toe.

2 Walk tall, moving freely from the hips, pushing off with the back foot, feet parallel, lift chest.

3 Sit tall and well back in the chair, base of spine supported. Have one foot forward, or ankles lightly crossed.

When practising the right way to stand and walk, try to wear medium heels, as your weight is then balanced more evenly over the entire foot, knees easy, neither sagging nor stiff.

The pelvis should now be level. Lift the chest and let the shoulders drop and remain level, too. Walk proudly, feeling tall and elegant rather than consciously pulling in tummy and seat. When the spine is in line breathing is deeper, but don't try to 'hold' a good position or you may walk stiffly – just 'feel' tall.

## Bend those knees!

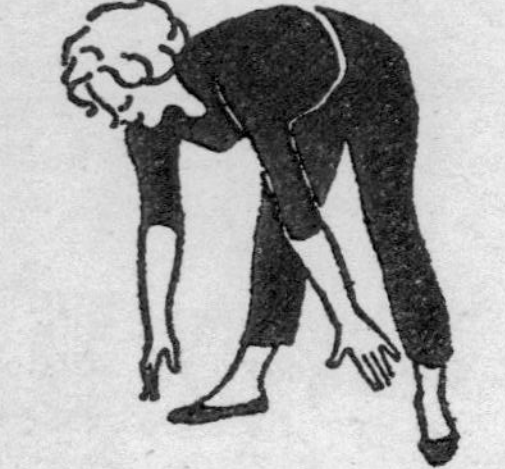

**1** Don't bend from waist with straight knees! It looks ugly and can cause strain and low backache.

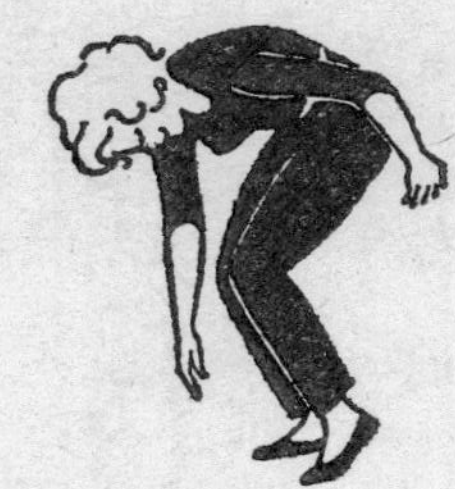

**2** Bend your knees when you touch your toes. Drop down with spine and knees relaxed, uncurl slowly and stand tall.

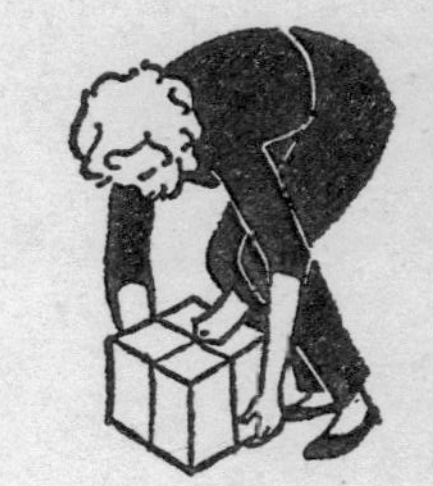

**3** Picking up a heavy weight – don't double up over it like this; bend knees with *straighter* back, head up, hips down.

It's a mistake to make our backs do all the work when the legs can help to take the strain. If you are lifting a heavy weight go down with the back as straight as possible, feet apart and close to it, push up with your leg muscles and the top of your head. Great care should be taken when lifting from the floor to think first and lift deliberately. As an exercise the relaxed drop down (2) and slow uncurling of the spine is a good movement to 'supple' and strengthen the back and, of course, the modern way to touch the toes.

## The 'stretchaway' – for midriff

Do the 'stretchaway' to counteract any tendency to 'slump' which can lead to a roll around the middle and on to middle-age spread! Stretch higher and higher – always trying to make one hand beat the other.

Placing the arms above the head and holding the position cannot have much effect; it is necessary to pull on the muscles of the midriff until you can feel them stretching harder and harder. Then and then only will you achieve a flat, smooth space between bust and hipline – a must for a good figure.

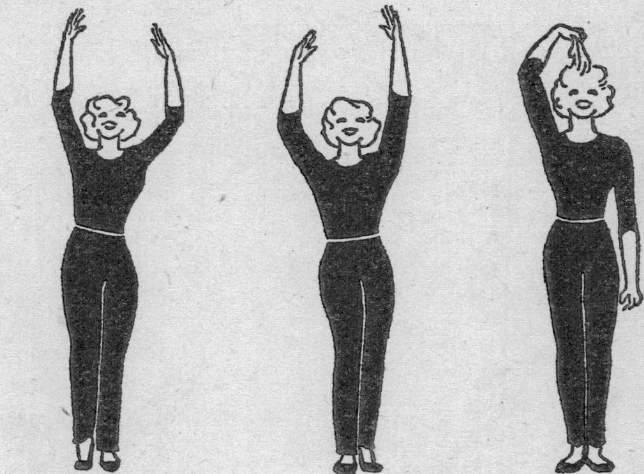

1 Raise right arm up sideways then left. Stretch up strongly towards ceiling with right.

2 Leaving right arm stretching upwards, stretch higher with left – then right and left again.

3 Stand as if being pulled up by your hair; try it to get the feeling of 'lift'.

**The 'rockaway'** – for feet and ankles

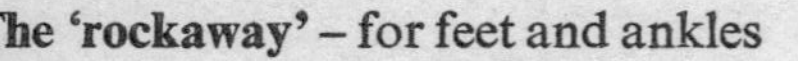

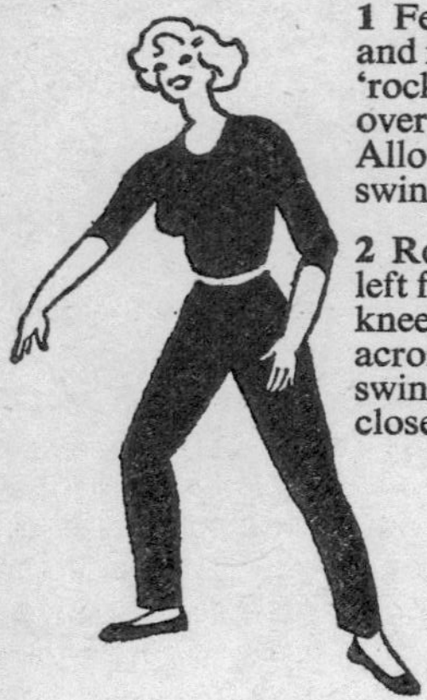

**1** Feet wide apart and relaxed knees, 'rock' your weight over right foot. Allow arms to swing with you.

**2** Rock back on to left foot, bending knees as weight goes across – arms swinging heavily, close to the body.

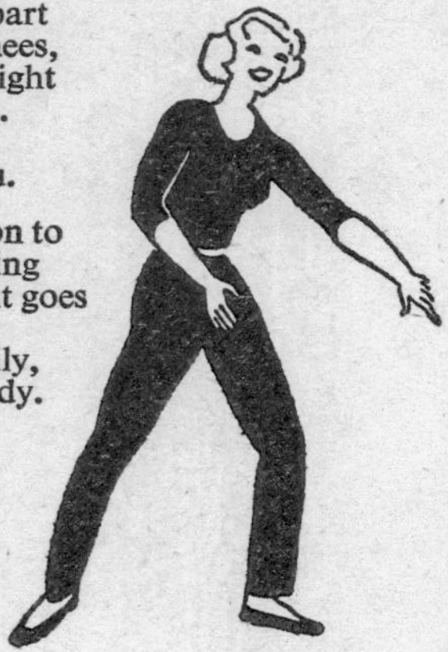

**3** Swing both arms high to right, weight over right foot, knee bent; clap lightly upwards – look at your hands.

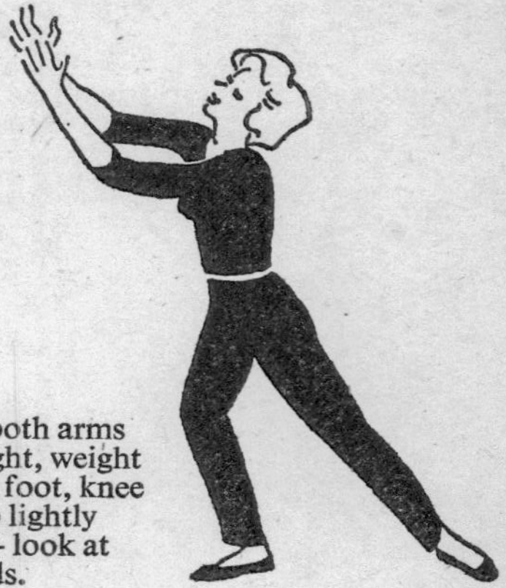

The classic 'change of weight' or 'rocking' movement is the basis of many exercises. To move to your fullest capacity you must have a wide stance and be able to change the weight from foot to foot. This is easily done by relaxing the knees throughout, with a deeper bend as the weight goes over and the arms swing like a pendulum. The movement is *down, up – down in the middle and up at the sides*. 'Feeling the floor' through the feet is one way of getting movement throughout the body as explained in 'How to practise,' page 16.

**'Swing around'** – waistline

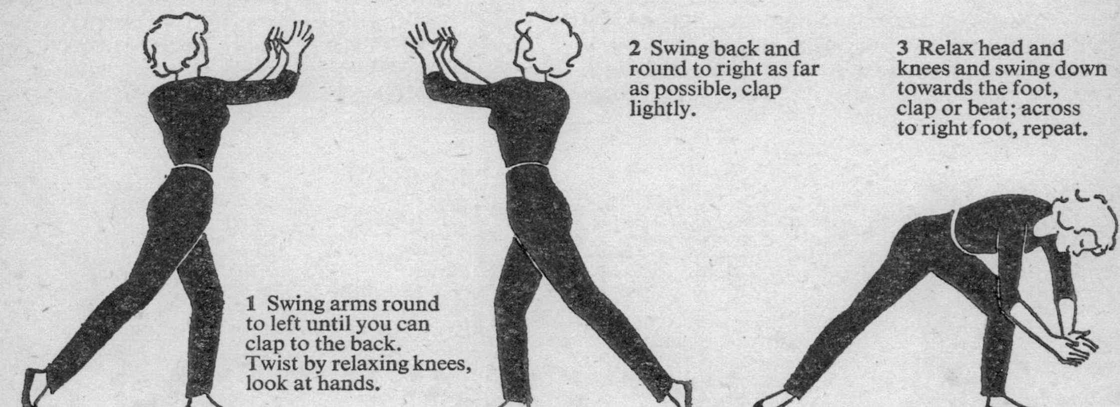

1 Swing arms round to left until you can clap to the back. Twist by relaxing knees, look at hands.

2 Swing back and round to right as far as possible, clap lightly.

3 Relax head and knees and swing down towards the foot, clap or beat; across to right foot, repeat.

The object of this exercise is to move in every possible direction. For a change from the clap, slip off your slippers (excellent for the feet!) and swing them round. Beat the soles together lightly.

'Swing and beat' can be done to several rhythms; the beat or clap accentuating the first beat of the second bar of music, the swing using the first bar.

Really try to get round as far as you can for the first part and to bend as low as possible for the second part.

## **'Reachaway'** – for waistline (slow tango time)

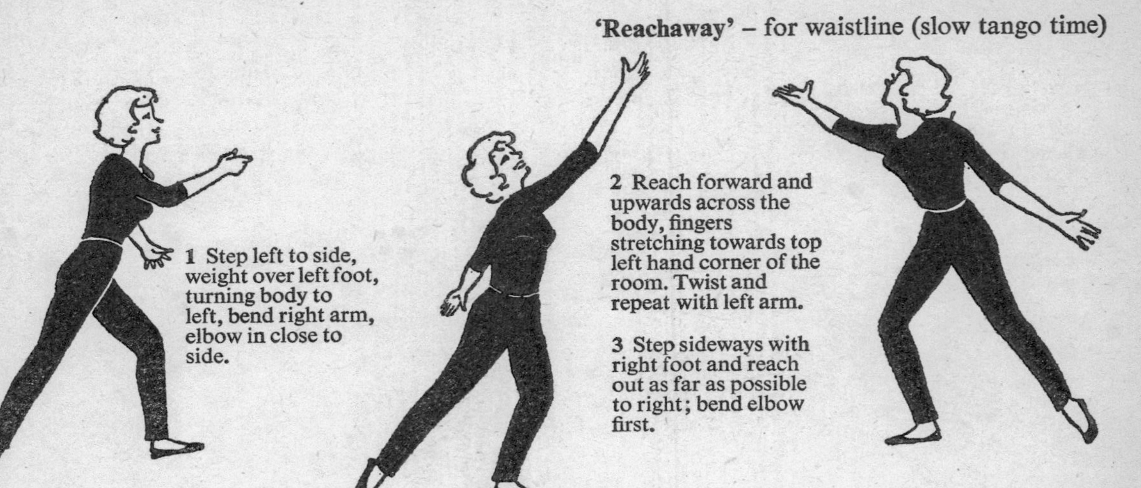

**1** Step left to side, weight over left foot, turning body to left, bend right arm, elbow in close to side.

**2** Reach forward and upwards across the body, fingers stretching towards top left hand corner of the room. Twist and repeat with left arm.

**3** Step sideways with right foot and reach out as far as possible to right; bend elbow first.

Use your rocking change of weight to reach out in every direction. Move more by reaching farther than ever before. It's the last inch of the stretch that helps to slim the waistline. The knee bend is a must, and the 'reachaway' must develop from a bent elbow before the arm straightens to the tips of the fingers. When you reach sideways, try to touch that wall! Remember, step, bend, reach – anywhere and everywhere, find a new direction every time.

## ‘Two-way stretch – for waistline (slow tango, waltz-time)

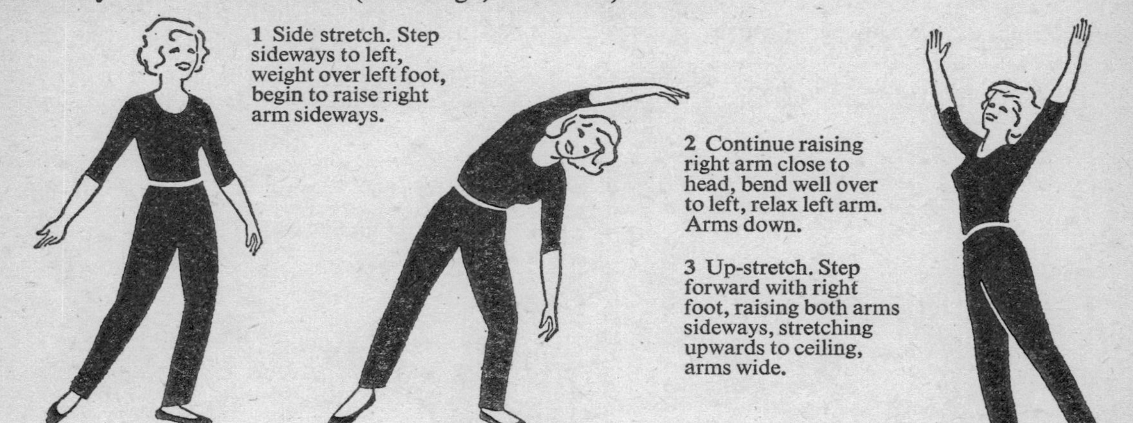

1 Side stretch. Step sideways to left, weight over left foot, begin to raise right arm sideways.

2 Continue raising right arm close to head, bend well over to left, relax left arm. Arms down.

3 Up-stretch. Step forward with right foot, raising both arms sideways, stretching upwards to ceiling, arms wide.

The main difference between the old and the new way to do this stretch movement is in the bend of the knee. The arm stretches up to the ceiling on its way overhead, but once there, a relaxed bounce of the knees takes the stiffness out of the movement. The top arm is then lowered as the weight is transferred to the right foot and the left arm comes up and over in the same way. 3. A straightforward lifting up of the arms, weight on front foot, a classical stretch and a nice finish.

## The 'skating swing' – for hipline (waltz-time or slow four)

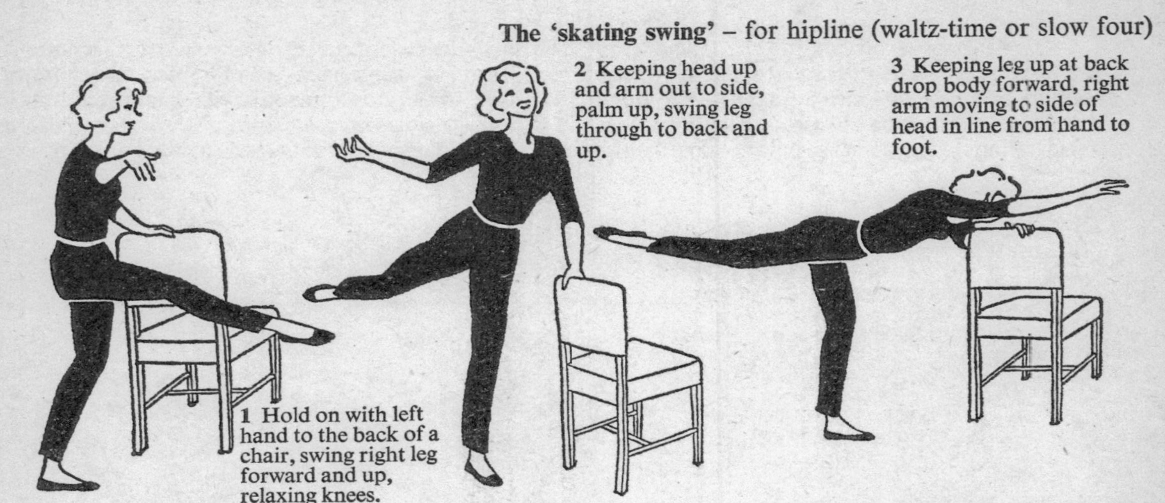

1 Hold on with left hand to the back of a chair, swing right leg forward and up, relaxing knees.

2 Keeping head up and arm out to side, palm up, swing leg through to back and up.

3 Keeping leg up at back drop body forward, right arm moving to side of head in line from hand to foot.

Start by swinging the leg forward and back only, with relaxed knees (1 and 2). This is the basic leg swing for hipline, simple and easy to do; it becomes an exercise if you swing seven times and change to the other leg on eight. The skating swing is excellent for tummy and back, as you can feel when you practise it. The muscles tighten and give a feeling of support to the body. This type of movement helps to fashion a natural corset of muscle, which gives a slimmer line to the figure.

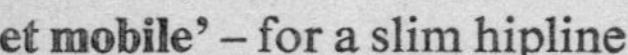

**'Get mobile'** – for a slim hipline

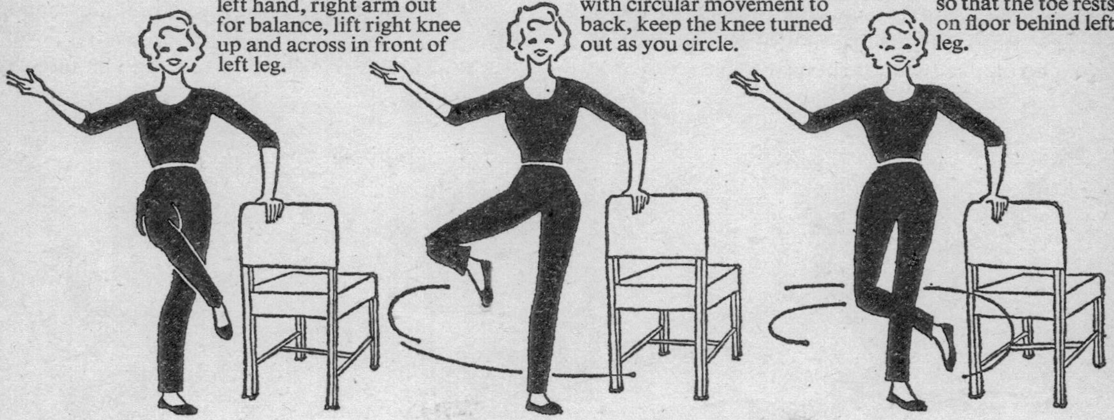

**1** Hold back of chair with left hand, right arm out for balance, lift right knee up and across in front of left leg.

**2** Swing right knee outwards with circular movement to back, keep the knee turned out as you circle.

**3** Drop toe to floor so that the toe rests on floor behind left leg.

Try to do this exercise every day, it will help to prevent the hips from widening or becoming stiff. It is similar to a ballet movement, but softer and more relaxed. Let the standing leg bend a little. As you take the outside knee across and round to the back, keep it turned out as much as possible, try not to let it drop as it circles to the back, rest it for a second lightly on the toe. Head up and pull up in the midriff, circle three times, then turn around and circle the other leg.

## 'Trim trio'

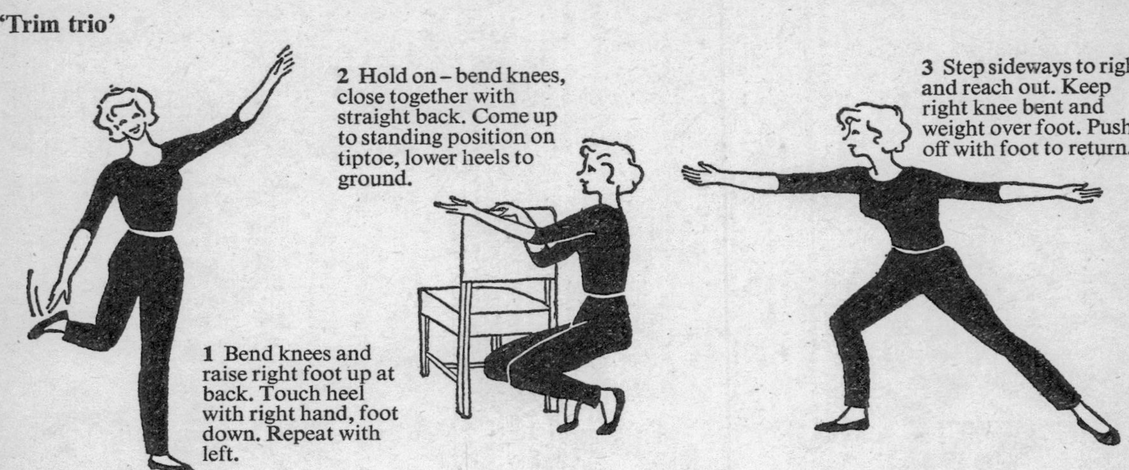

**1** Bend knees and raise right foot up at back. Touch heel with right hand, foot down. Repeat with left.

**2** Hold on – bend knees, close together with straight back. Come up to standing position on tiptoe, lower heels to ground.

**3** Step sideways to right and reach out. Keep right knee bent and weight over foot. Push off with foot to return.

Three combination movements. 1. Heel-touching, if practised regularly, will help to slim hips and neaten seat. Do it all round the room, to the radio.

The deep knee bend (2) works on hip, thigh and back. Try to get hips well down when practising. Don't overdo it. Finish by walking round the room on tiptoe.

3. A lunging movement well known for grace and good posture, also strengthens legs and back. Hold position for a few seconds and then come back to 'standing tall'.

## 'Spinal curl'

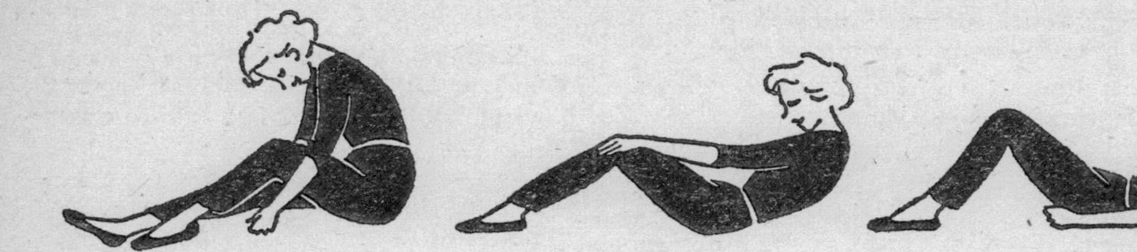

**1** Sit on floor with relaxed knees. Curl forward over them, 'letting go' deliberately, back rounded.

**2** Roll back, gradually uncurling and leaving head until last, arms drop to sides, allow hands to relax.

**3** Flatten out, relax until you feel that your back is sinking into the floor, leaving no 'daylight' or space between.

Perhaps the most simple and natural movement to flatten the tummy is to lie down and sit up, without helping yourself to do so. If the muscles have become slack and you find this difficult at first, slip both hands under you, palms downward on the floor.

This will raise you up easily. It is important to practise this movement because it is part of many abdominal sequences and a base for other floor exercises. Also, when this becomes easy you are on the way to fashioning your figure – if you eat sensibly as well.

**'Jolly along'** – to counteract weight below the waist

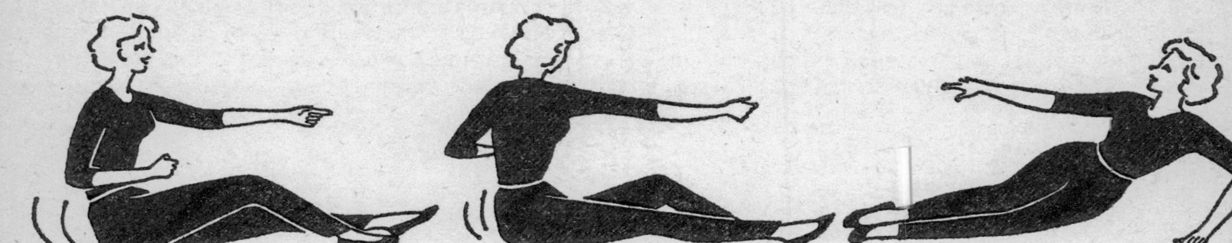

**1** Sit on floor, extend left arm and leg, lifting left hip, and move forward one pace.

**2** Stretch right arm and leg forward and move forward again, lifting right hip. Repeat backwards.

**3** Rock your weight over and on to the left hip and hand, feet together, look back at right hand.

These are fun to do to music and certainly help to break down surplus weight on hips, seat and tummy. It's easy to 'thicken' in these areas and some well tried floor exercises can be very useful. Do them in with your housework or at an odd moment when you are 'dressed for the part.'

You could follow up the hip walk (1 and 2) by the 'Rock and Roll' (3) to the same tempo.

Add a complete roll over on to the tummy, face downwards – very energetic but good for the figure!

## **'Twist and rock'** – waistline and tummy muscles



**1** Roll over onto left hip and hand. Take right knee over and across to touch the floor; repeat to other side.

**2** Sit on floor, ankles crossed, hands at sides. Touch left knee with right elbow. Return to starting position. Repeat to other side.

Tummy exercises with a twist can help to whittle the waistline, too.

1. A progression from the last exercise, the basic rock and roll. Get used to this first, then rock further still and bring the knee well over to touch the floor.

2. Elbow to knee, will go to the same rhythm, so these can be joined to make a short sequence.

3. This is still stronger for toning up tummy muscles. Not hard to do, because the momentum caused by rocking back helps you to lift both legs up without strain. As you lower legs to floor, keep them easy and touch toes lightly with one hand.

**3** Sit tall, knees relaxed. Rock back onto hands, raise legs from floor and tap sides of feet lightly together. Lower to floor.

## 'Swing and snap'

Here is a full body movement excellent for thighs and tummy and the figure generally. Get contrast by relaxing as you swing down and up but stretch strongly at the finish.

The 'snap' is made with the thumb and middle finger, a current movement which emphasizes rhythm, often used in modern singing and dancing.

Most important is the double knee bend as you swing down and then up. Without this, the movement is stiff and of less value.

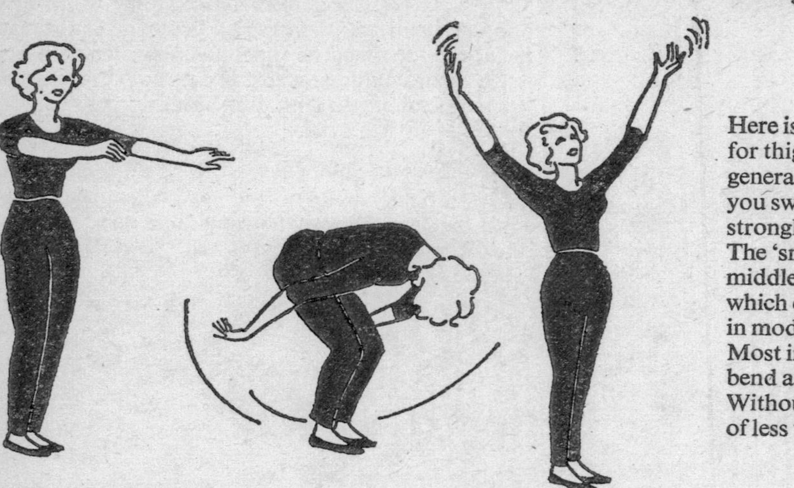

**1** Stand tall with both arms stretched forward at shoulder level, knees easy, ready to relax as you swing down.

**2** Relax head and knees, swing down, curling the spine, arms following through to back.

**3** Bend knees again as arms and body swing up to full height, stretch arms high, snap fingers twice.

**'Beauty spot' exercises** – neater necklines: waltz-time

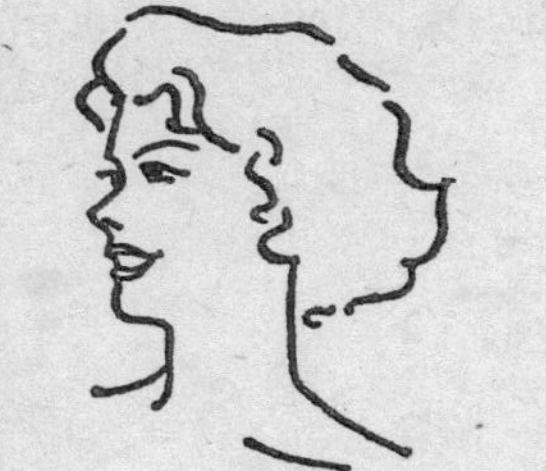

**1** Turn head slowly to right until chin is in line with shoulders, keep movement easy. Face front.

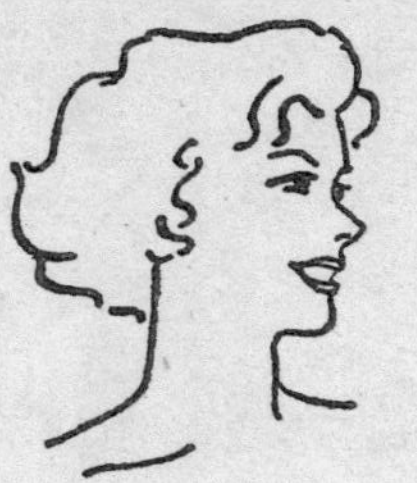

**2** Turn head to left, try to see over shoulder, but don't force head round; keep shoulders relaxed. Face front.

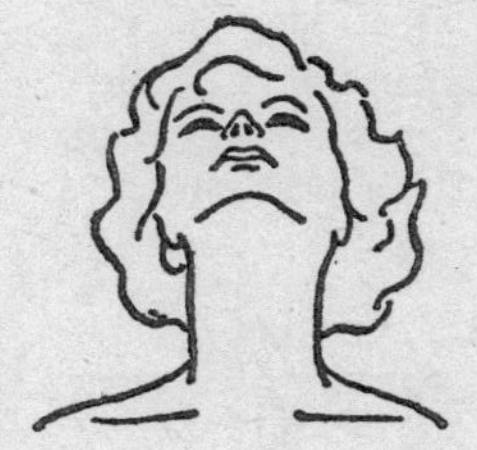

**3** Raise chin and let head drop back gently, looking up at ceiling. Open and close mouth, drop your chin.

For a youthful appearance, never neglect the neck. It is essential to keep the head turning freely and to tone up the muscles of the throat. Do these head movements whenever you can and, in addition, allow the head to circle gently round in both directions.

Apart from helping to keep a clean chin and jaw, moving this way has a relaxing effect, relieves tension at the back of the neck and helps to counteract the effect of a dropped position of the head, which occurs when doing jobs below eye level.

## **'Beauty spot' exercises** – 'slim and shapely' for shoulders and upper arms: slow foxtrot

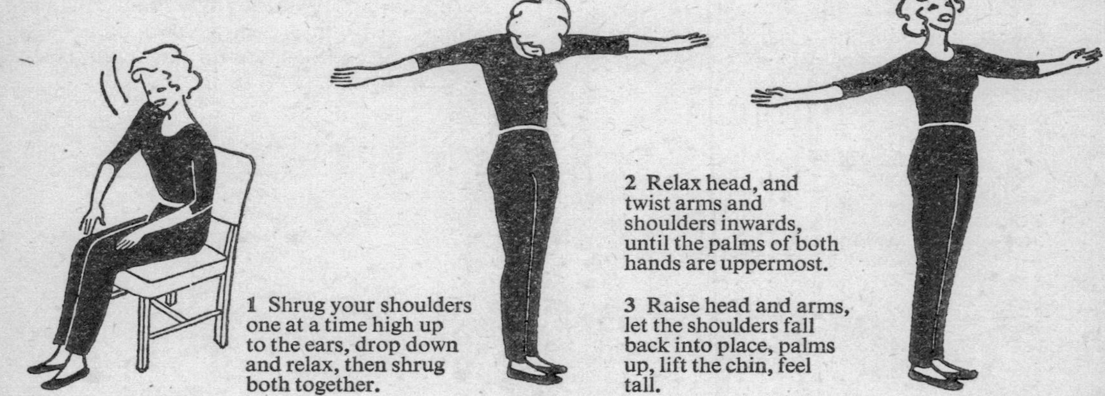

1 Shrug your shoulders one at a time high up to the ears, drop down and relax, then shrug both together.

2 Relax head, and twist arms and shoulders inwards, until the palms of both hands are uppermost.

3 Raise head and arms, let the shoulders fall back into place, palms up, lift the chin, feel tall.

Shapely shoulders and slim upper arms are a great asset, and worth a little effort to maintain. Shoulders should be kept moving to prevent them getting 'set' – thick through – or rounded. They are a focal point and need to be straight and supple. These exercises will help to keep them slim and mobile. Shrug your shoulders, then roll them around backwards in small circles. You will feel the top of the chest and upper back moving too. The twist (2 & 3) will help to slim upper arms; screw them round gently – you will feel them tightening where they need it most.

## **'Skipalong'** – for Back beauty

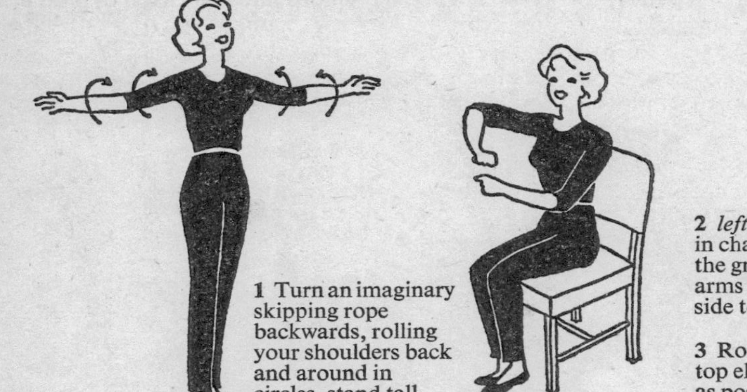

1 Turn an imaginary skipping rope backwards, rolling your shoulders back and around in circles, stand tall, head up.

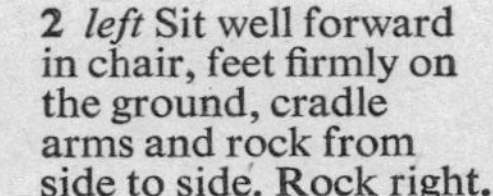

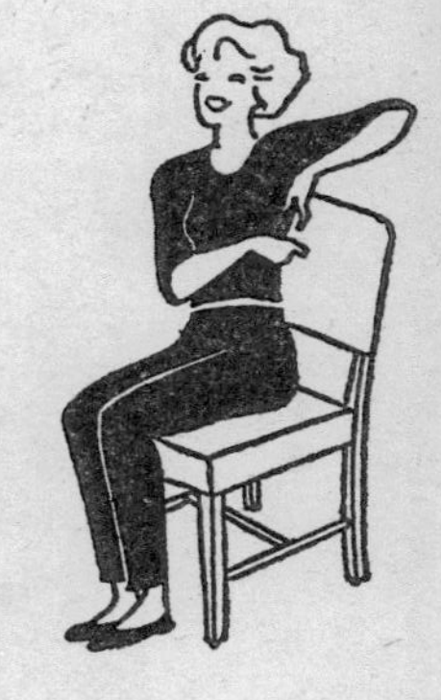

2 *left* Sit well forward in chair, feet firmly on the ground, cradle arms and rock from side to side. Rock right.

3 Rock left, lifting the top elbow up as high as possible. Exaggerate slightly, head up.

When you 'skip', try to feel real movement in shoulders and upper back. Excellent for Dowager's hump! Lift as you circle shoulders and wrists.

'Skip' first, then 'rock the baby', doing both movements several times, dropping arms on count of eight. Now stand up to skip, feet together and bending knees for a bouncy effect. Step to side, so that feet are apart for rocking the baby. Music should be steady but not heavy, eight melody notes to the bar as in 'Nola', light and gay.

(Suggested music: 'Nola')

## Bustline beauty

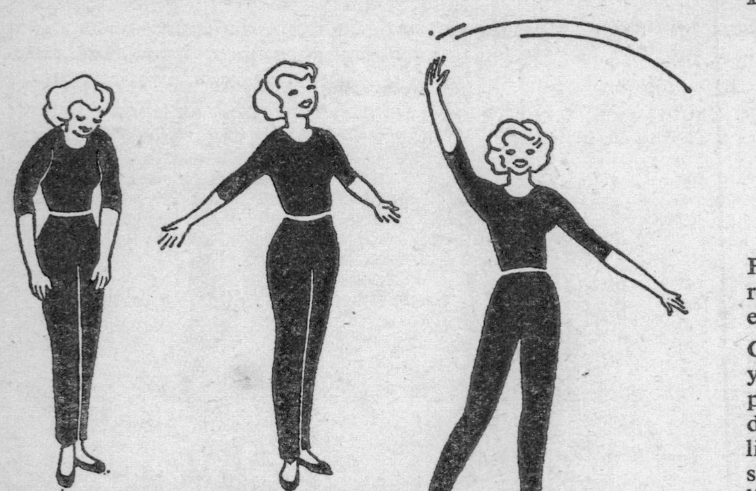

1 Relax head, shoulders and arms, palms down, as you breathe out to expel all used up air from lungs.

2 Lift the head and chest as you breathe in, rolling the shoulders and arms back and down, palms facing front.

3 Weight on left foot, circle right arm across, up and round, stretching up at peak of circle, repeat with left.

For a pretty bustline, lift the chest and relax the shoulders. Good posture is essential.

Get the deep breathing habit to help you. First, empty the lungs; note the position, (1) rounded shoulders, dropped head. Breathe in slowly, lifting the head and chest, relaxing the shoulders (2). Result, a lovely uplifted line. Continue the 'lift' by stepping sideways and circling the arms alternately (3). Reach high as you circle to stretch the waistline and lift the bust. (Music: Waltz-time)

## **Swim** – for curves

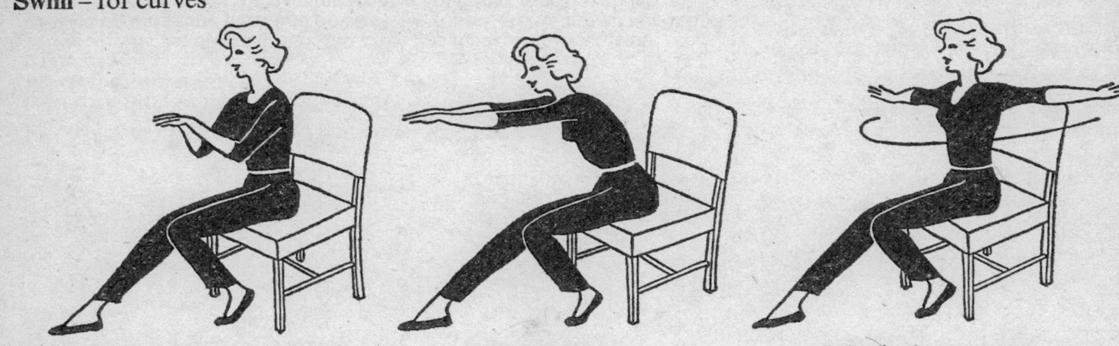

1 Sit well forward on chair, one knee bent, one straight. Hands together at chest level, palms downwards, thumbs touching.

2 Push both arms strongly forward, weight over knee, lean forward as far as possible.

3 Bring both arms out to side, as in breast-stroke, back straight, shoulders relaxed.

Another way to gain prettier curves is to develop the chest by swimming. The rhythmical action strengthens the muscles that matter. Try the movements sitting or standing. 'Swim' slowly and gracefully as if you were cleaving your way through the water.

Add an alternate arm circling movement similar to backstroke. It will help to build up the bustline and slim the waist.

Go swimming as well whenever possible, but a 'daily dozen' strokes on dry land are well worth the time and effort. (Music: slow four-time)

## Fascinating fingers

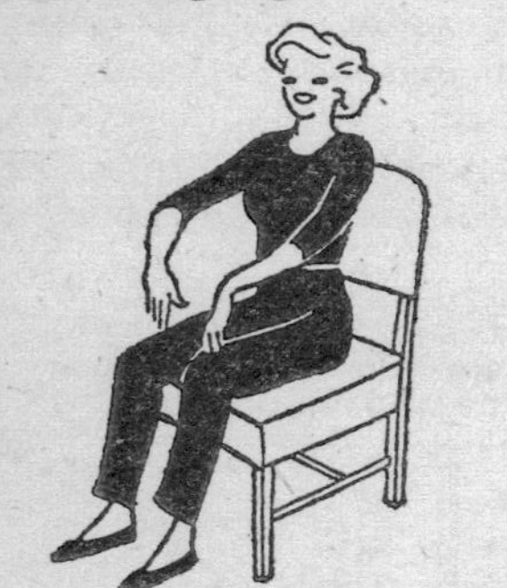

1 Sit with arms relaxed, lift hands, wrists up, and touch both knees with fingertips, stretching wrists.

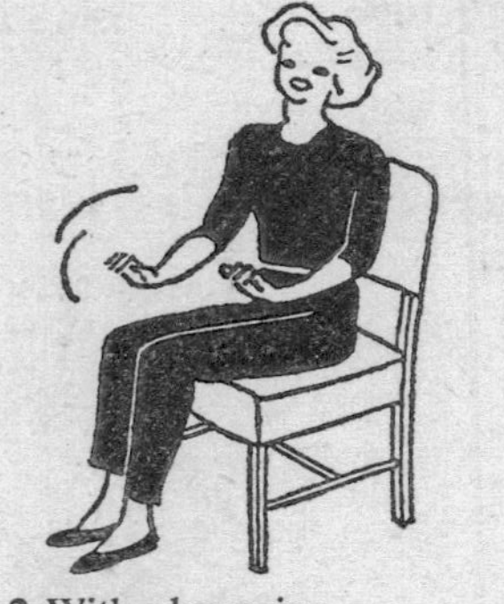

2 With a bouncing movement turn fingers up and stretch wrists down to touch knees.

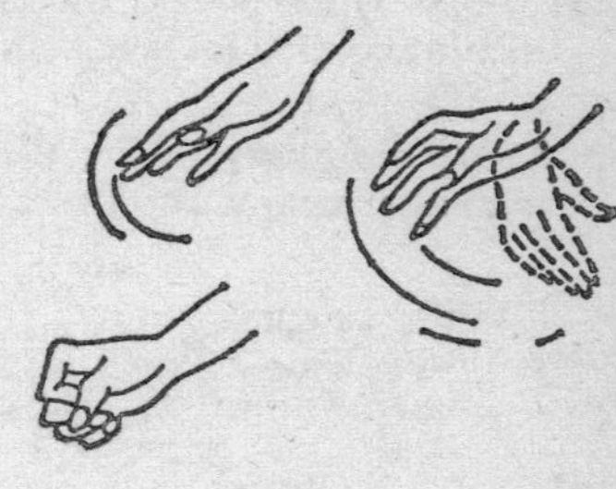

3 Make a tight fist, then open hands and stretch fingers strongly. Shake hands downwards from the wrist.

Pretty hands can fascinate. Their size and shape are relatively unimportant, the secret lies in the way in which they are used.

First, they must be supple, so follow these movements. (1) Touch your knees with fingertips, stretching the wrist; lift the fingers and stretch the wrists down to touch the knees. (2) Repeat, making both movements bigger as you go along.

To keep fingers slim and supple, see (3). Clench and unclench the hands, then shake to relax. (Music can be tango, foxtrot or waltz)

**'Toes up'** – for pretty feet

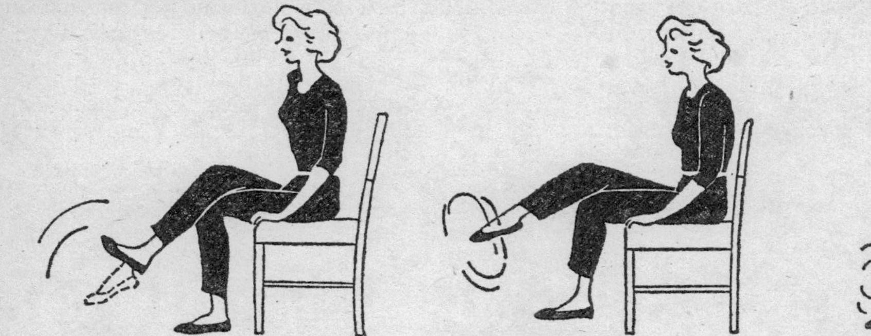

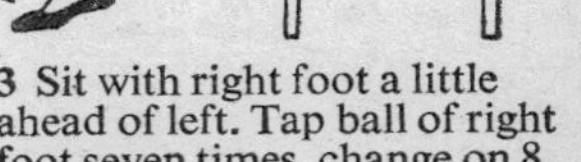

**1** Sit; cross right leg over left. Bend and stretch right foot up and down for six counts, change on 7 and 8; repeat.

**2** Circle right foot from ankle, seven times; on the count of eight change to other leg.

**3** Sit with right foot a little ahead of left. Tap ball of right foot seven times, change on 8.

Let your feet out whenever you can! Slip off your shoes and give your feet a chance to relax. See that stockings are long enough in the foot and that your feet are restricted as little as possible.

Keep them supple. 'Solid' feet without 'spring' are seldom youthful. Move them around with these exercises whenever you have a minute to spare.

In (1) the toes turn up to meet the nose! bending and stretching the instep. (2 and 3) Circle and tap them and keep the ankles easy and slender. Walk around on tiptoe. (Music for this: Happy Feet)

## **Stretch and let go** – for relaxation

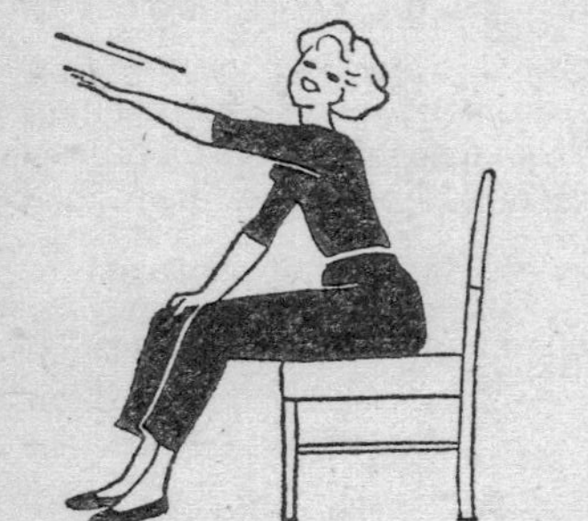

1 Stretch out one arm strongly in front, tensing muscles from shoulder to fingertips. Hold it, while you count five.

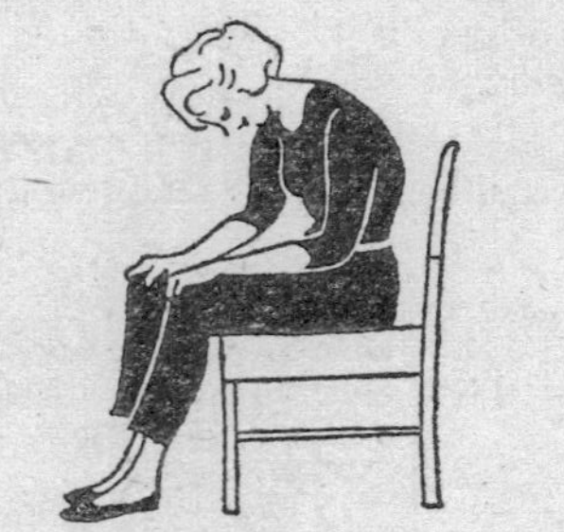

2 Relax the arm and mentally let go so that it drops and flops into your lap. Repeat with other arm.

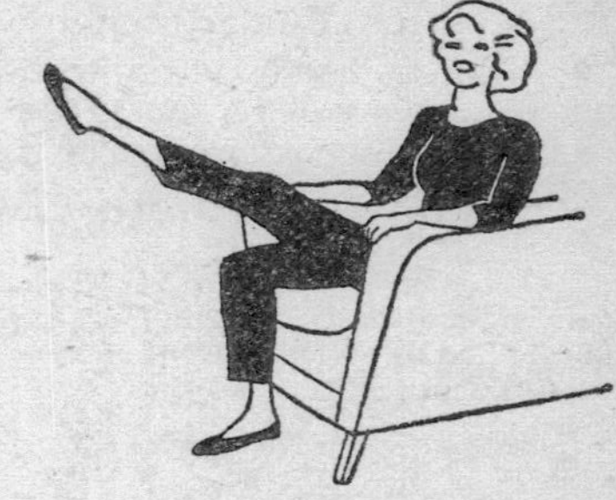

3 Raise one leg and stretch out, tensing and pointing toes. Relax, letting leg drop to floor; repeat with other leg.

When learning to relax it is necessary first of all to know when you are tense, to consciously recognize that you are keyed up or nervously exhausted. Then and then only can you find a way to counteract tension, and to let go completely.

These movements are intended as an introduction, a means of getting the feeling of muscular tension and relaxation. Follow them and you will get contrast between strain and rest.

To unwind mentally, try to see nothing but black velvet, everywhere.

## Fighting fatigue

**1** Lie on floor with bent knees, hands loosely at sides. Relax them back into the floor, leaving no space.

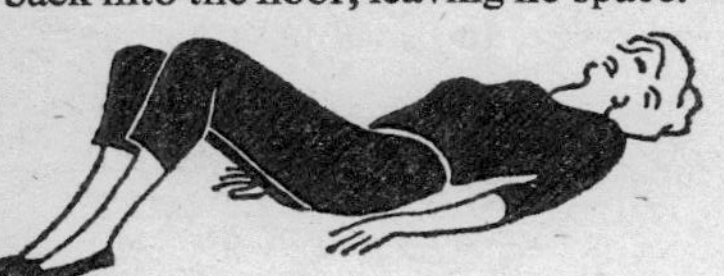

Relaxing flat on the floor with feet up will help to renew your energy. Lying this way is infinitely more restful than sitting with feet on the floor. It will allow the blood to flow more freely into your face, renewing the cells, refreshing you in a short space of time.

Lie as in (1). Try to feel that you are so heavy that you will sink through the floor! Stay this way for ten minutes, then slowly get back into circulation by doing the simple leg exercise (3). It's good for the tummy as well.

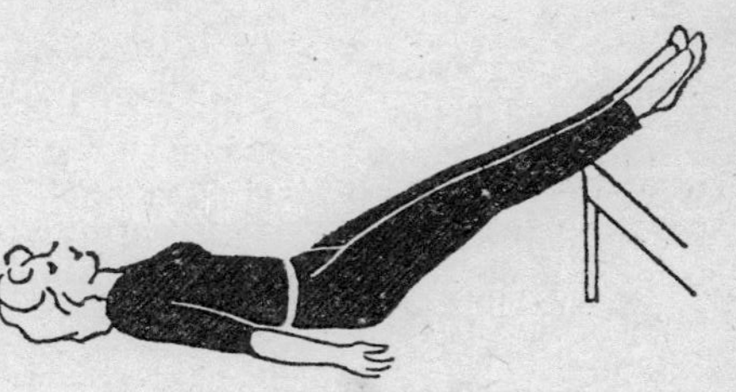

**2** Lie flat on floor with feet up on seat of a soft chair. If chair surface is hard, use a cushion.

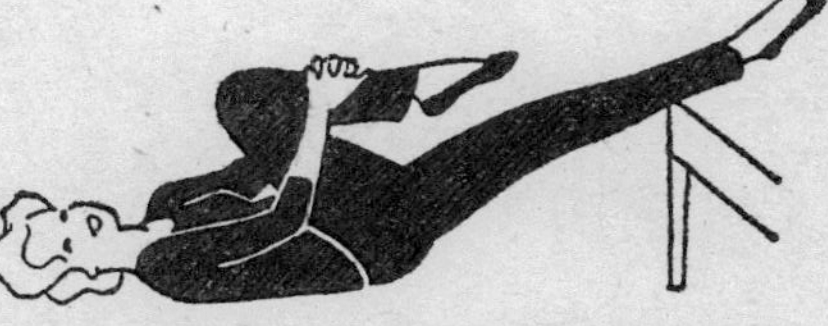

**3** Pull one leg up as close to chest as possible, put back on chair and relax. Repeat with other knee.

## Fireside flop

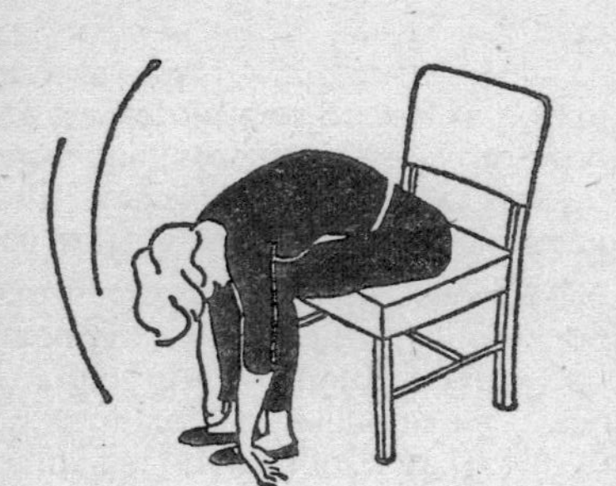

**1** Sit and relax, letting go completely; drop down over your knees with hands flopping on the floor, head down.

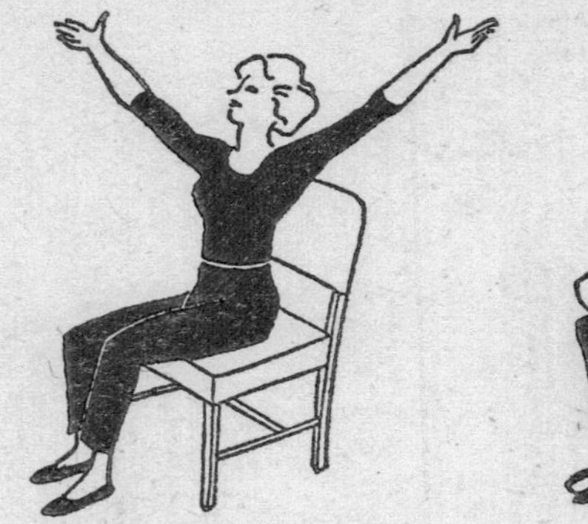

**2** Slowly uncurl the spine, sit up, stretch arms above head, keep on stretching up until you yawn.

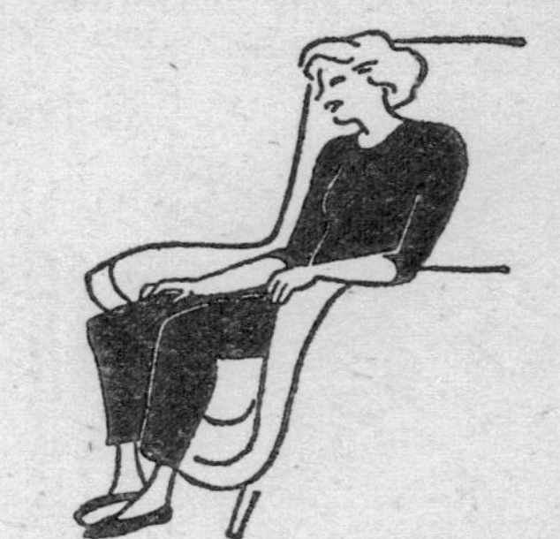

**3** Let arms flop down to a comfortable position. Relax your hands, feet up if possible; go completely limp.

To induce a feeling of real relaxation try to make yourself yawn. Flop and stretch as shown here, giving yourself time to slow down. The steady unrolling and stretching movements are excellent for the spine. They help to keep the back strong and supple, aiding good posture.

Be sure to keep warm; even a low stool placed beneath your feet will help rest you. Training yourself to relax takes time, but persevere until you get the cat-nap habit. Those who do so awake truly refreshed and able to cope once more.

## In the home

Learning to move the Keep Fit way is of tremendous help with the housework. The every day actions shown on this page are easier to do and kinder to the figure when good movement becomes automatic.

(1) Using a sweeper or mop is not tiring if done rhythmically, learning to relax the knees. (2) Take advantage of every reaching up movement you make to slim your waistline as you work, and counteract slump; stretch up as high as you can from the waist.
(3) Bending your knees instead of stooping will save your back and makes you more graceful.

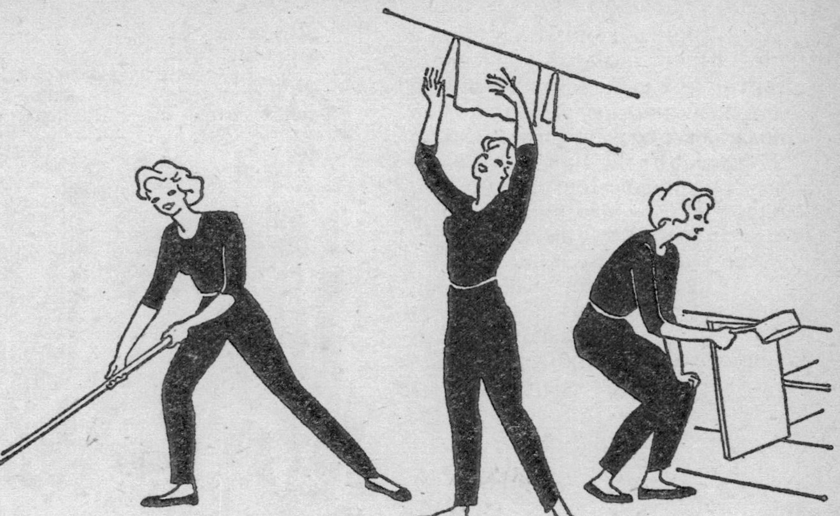

**1** When using the vacuum cleaner or mop, relax knees and change weight from foot to foot.

**2** Reach high to airing line or top shelf, best foot forward, and stretch from waistline.

**3** Bend knees first as you go down; push up head first, legs doing most of the work.

## Good balance

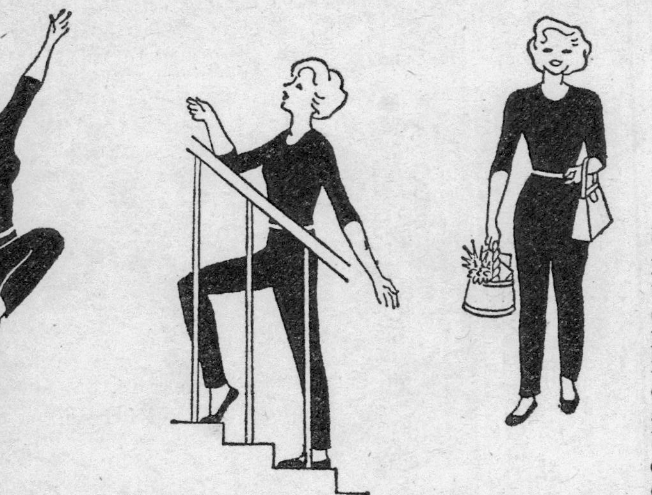

**1** Stand on one leg to put on slippers. Head up and lift the foot high – stretch top arm.

**2** Ignore the handrail when you go upstairs – head up and keep a straight line from head to foot.

**3** When shopping distribute the load equally in either hand; change from side to side frequently.

(1) Good balance helps posture. Train your muscles to support you by standing to put on your slippers.

(2) Make your staircase part of your home gymnasium. Don't lean forward or drag yourself up. Come down and go up as if you were making an entrance and exit. Push off from the back foot and move smoothly upwards; come down carefully and upright.

(3) Don't let a loaded basket pull you down on one side, or clutch your handbag under one arm with shoulder raised. Don't grip your handbag – hold it firmly, but without tension.

## Brush swing – circulation

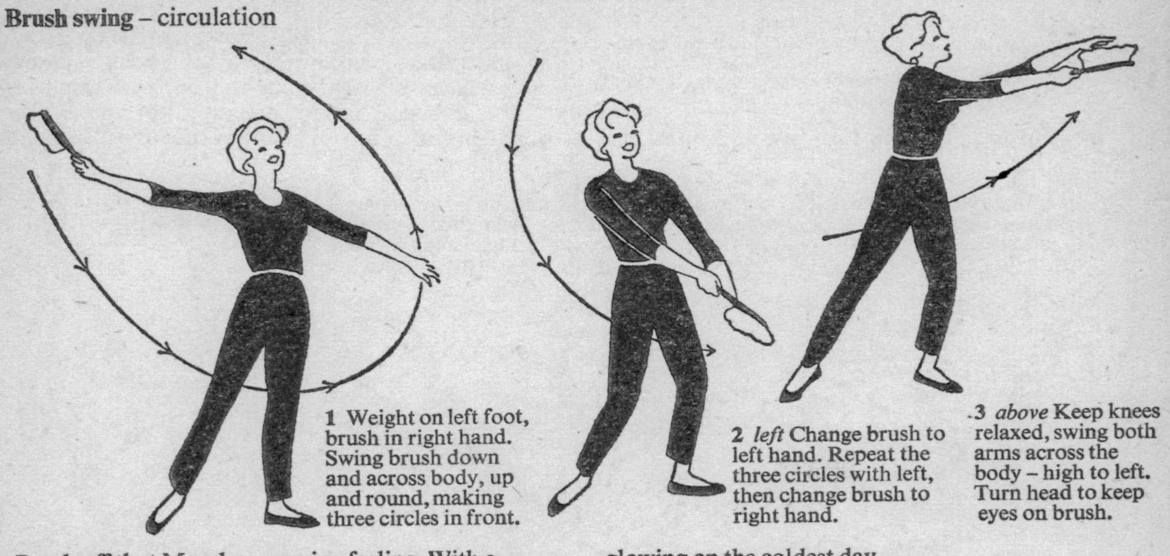

1 Weight on left foot, brush in right hand. Swing brush down and across body, up and round, making three circles in front.

2 *left* Change brush to left hand. Repeat the three circles with left, then change brush to right hand.

3 *above* Keep knees relaxed, swing both arms across the body – high to left. Turn head to keep eyes on brush.

Brush off that Monday morning feeling. With a minute or two to spare and a steady waltz on record or radio, pick up a brush and swing it to get you glowing on the coldest day.

The brush will add a little weight to the swings and help to lift the bustline as you reach up.

**Brush swing** – continued

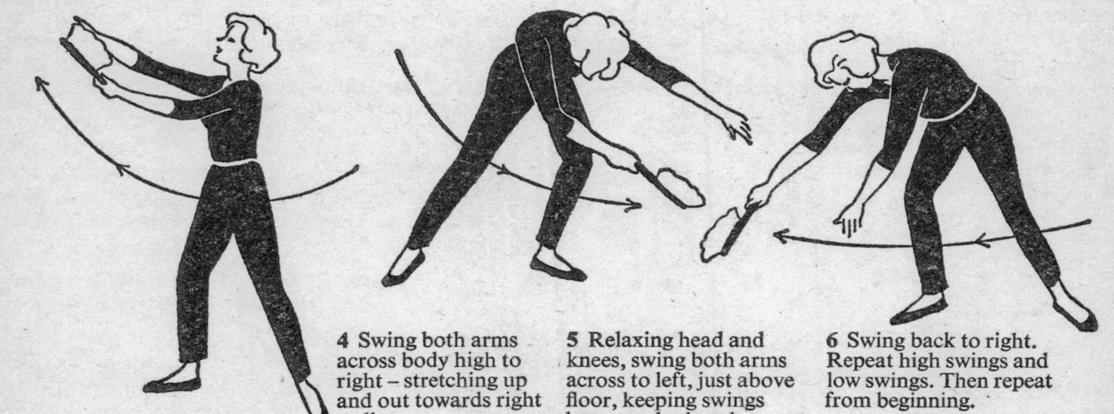

**4** Swing both arms across body high to right – stretching up and out towards right wall.

**5** Relaxing head and knees, swing both arms across to left, just above floor, keeping swings heavy and relaxed.

**6** Swing back to right. Repeat high swings and low swings. Then repeat from beginning.

Circle with a slightly relaxed arm but stretch up to the ceiling at the top of the circle: chest, back and shoulders will benefit from this. The low swing (5) should be kept heavy and relaxed like the swing of the pendulum of a clock.

Reach out to the walls as you swing and bend your knees.

(Music: Waltz-time – 16 bars)

## Teenage trimmers – waistline

If you want a wasp waist, practise all three movements gracefully and without hurrying because in each case the position is 'held' for a second or two.

In (1) bend well over to 'see' that your toe is pointed.

(2) and (3) feels slightly acrobatic, but it is easy to do, and is a perfect side stretch, if done well. Return to sitting position and do three times before rolling over to sit on your other side.

(4) is simple, but depends for results on really relaxed knees and a good twist.

(Music: Waltz-time)

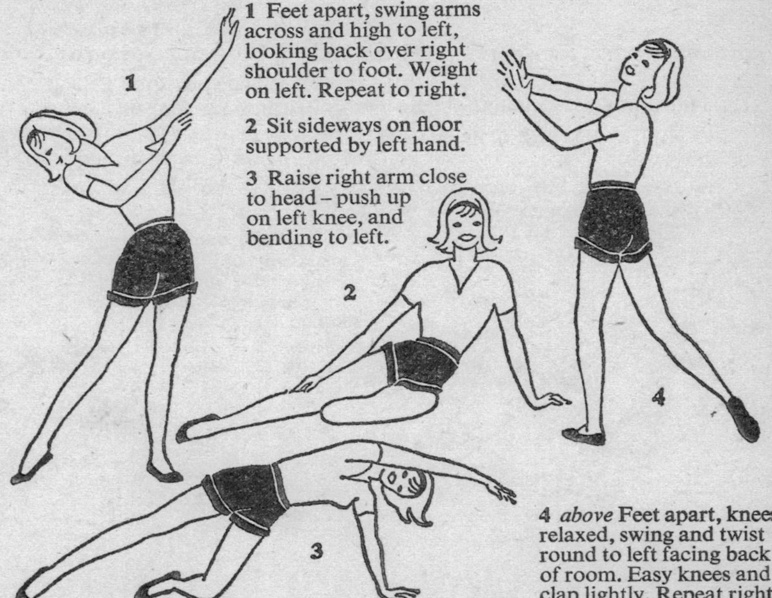


1 Feet apart, swing arms across and high to left, looking back over right shoulder to foot. Weight on left. Repeat to right.

2 Sit sideways on floor supported by left hand.

3 Raise right arm close to head – push up on left knee, and bending to left.

4 *above* Feet apart, knees relaxed, swing and twist round to left facing back of room. Easy knees and clap lightly. Repeat right.

## Teenage Trimmers – tummy muscles

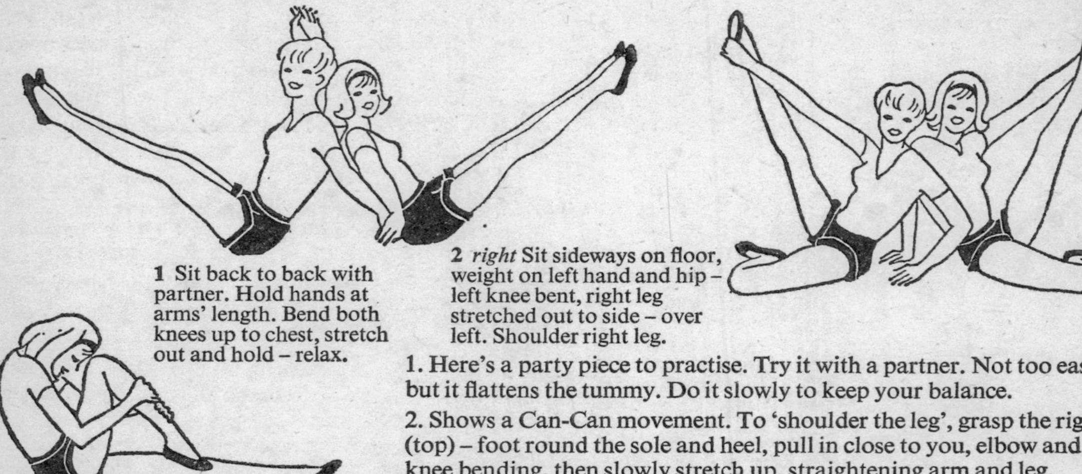

**1** Sit back to back with partner. Hold hands at arms' length. Bend both knees up to chest, stretch out and hold – relax.

**2** *right* Sit sideways on floor, weight on left hand and hip – left knee bent, right leg stretched out to side – over left. Shoulder right leg.

**3** Sit tall, feet together, knees relaxed. Grasp right knee and pull up to touch forehead. Lower leg, sit tall. Repeat left.

1. Here's a party piece to practise. Try it with a partner. Not too easy but it flattens the tummy. Do it slowly to keep your balance.

2. Shows a Can-Can movement. To 'shoulder the leg', grasp the right – (top) – foot round the sole and heel, pull in close to you, elbow and knee bending, then slowly stretch up, straightening arm and leg. Relax both and change sides.

To make exercises easy, get used to pulling the knee high and close to you. 3 will show you how.

(Music: Can-Can)

**Everybody dance** – hip and thigh

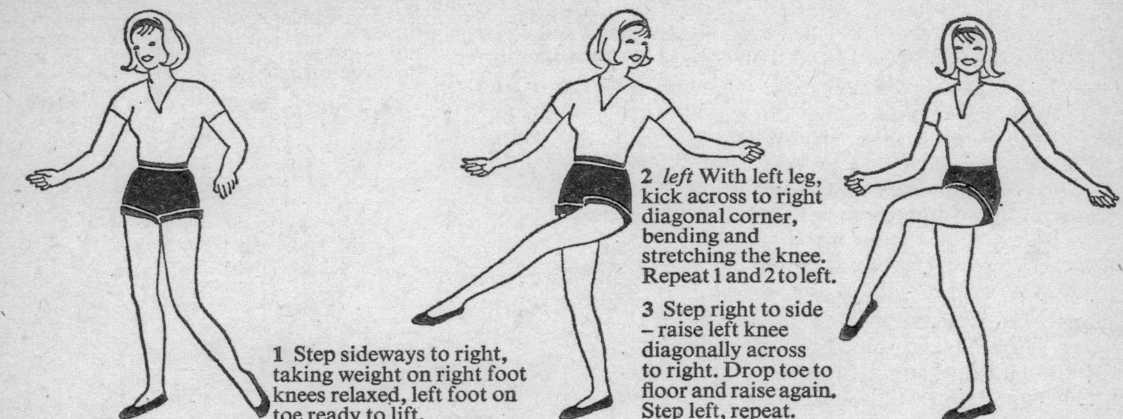

**1** Step sideways to right, taking weight on right foot knees relaxed, left foot on toe ready to lift.

**2** *left* With left leg, kick across to right diagonal corner, bending and stretching the knee. Repeat 1 and 2 to left.

**3** Step right to side – raise left knee diagonally across to right. Drop toe to floor and raise again. Step left, repeat.

Dancing the modern way is fine for feet and legs, hips and thighs, too. 1 & 2. Steps with a 'lift' help to keep the hipline slim and elegant.

If you have a sitting-down job – get busy with these. Step and kick across in the modern mood, snapping your fingers and kicking higher and higher.

Do the double knee lift – 3 – quite fast, pulling your tummy in as the knee comes up – (the modern contraction), and if you are a dancer, decide now never to give it up!

(Music: Madison or modern beat)

## **Sky high** – midriff and bustline

Watch that midriff! An unconscious slouch or slump can result in a roll and ruin the line between bust and hip. It should be supple, slender, long and flat. So the sky is the limit for stretching!

1. Relax first. 2. Slowly and strongly push the roof up and off until you ache in the middle. Follow it up by arm circling for bustline – see Brush Swing, page 87 – but lift against more resistance by picking up a book weighing 2 lb (1 kg). (3).

(Music: Waltz-time)

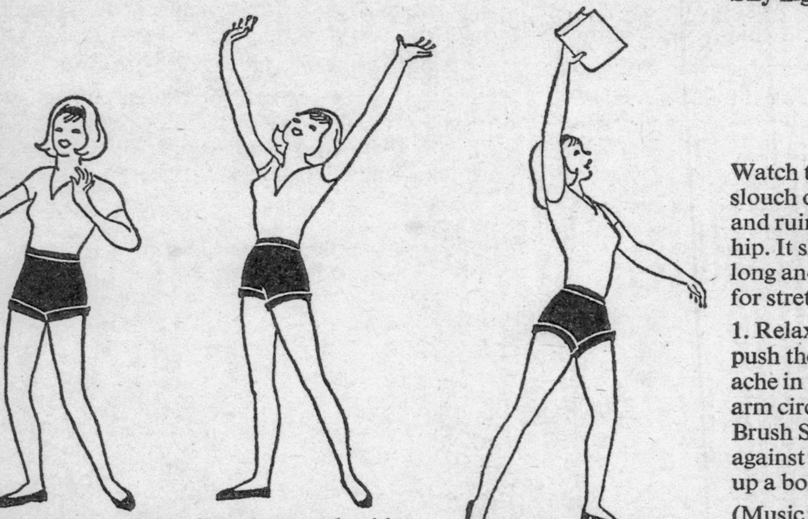

**1** Step sideways to right, relaxing knees and bringing hands up to shoulder height, palms up.

**2** Push upwards with palms towards ceiling, straighten knees and lift from the waistline; arms down sideways.

**3** Pick up a book or similar object – hold loosely, swing it up and around in circles, lifting at peak of swing.

## Exercise sequences – beat and clap – warm-up or introductory

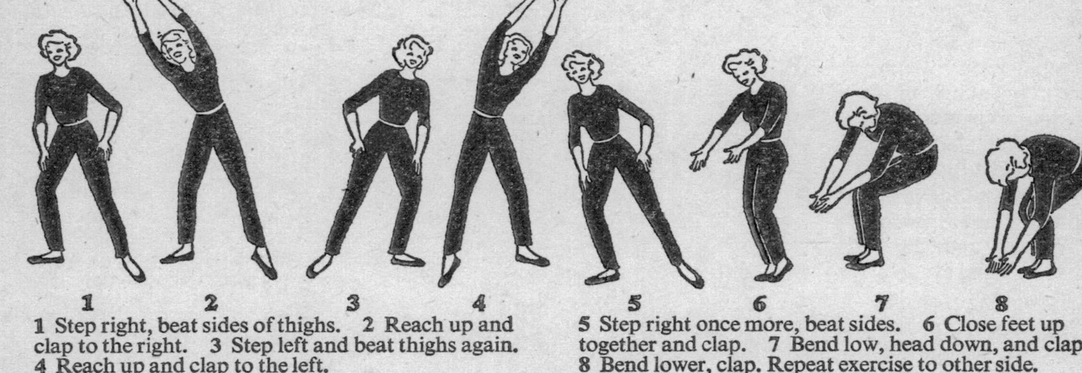


1 Step right, beat sides of thighs. 2 Reach up and clap to the right. 3 Step left and beat thighs again. 4 Reach up and clap to the left.

5 Step right once more, beat sides. 6 Close feet up together and clap. 7 Bend low, head down, and clap. 8 Bend lower, clap. Repeat exercise to other side.

Beat the sides lightly (i.e. slap with palm of hand) and stretch as you clap. Make sure your weight is over the correct foot and don't let your head poke forward. Reach up and give a bouncing clap, feeling the stretch at the waistline. Relax when you clap down towards the floor.

This takes 4 bars of music only, but repeated makes 8.

Try to set a suitable movement yourself to the next 8 bars. It could be a step and kick or some movement where the arms are at rest. Now you have used 16 bars, so repeat from the beginning to fill out a 32-bar chorus.

(Music: 'Ain't we got fun', or Slow foxtrot, waltz-time or tango. 8 bars)

**Knees up!** – a hip activity

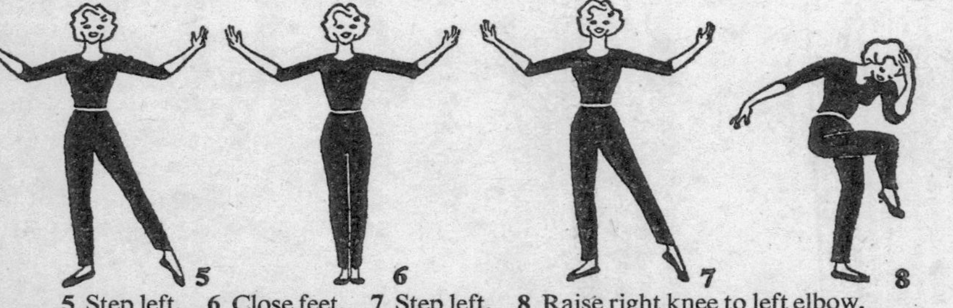


1 Step on to left foot. 2 Raise right knee. 3 Step on to right foot. 4 Raise left knee. (Repeat bringing knees up 8 times in all)

5 Step left. 6 Close feet. 7 Step left. 8 Raise right knee to left elbow. (Repeat to right, then left, and right again)

You can do this Sequence by yourself or with a partner.

Step slightly to the side first, then bring the knee up and slightly across – it's prettier than straight up – and remember to point the toe downwards.

Be sure to stand tall and keep your head up, because this strengthens back muscles and improves balance.

Touching the knee with the opposite elbow is quite simple as it's a fairly quick rhythm. You are soon away and stepping sideways again.

(Music: 'Cock of the North.' 16 bars)

## Fireside Twist – tummy muscles

You will find that it is much easier to sit tall for this exercise if you relax your knees and cross your ankles.

Pull up from the base of the spine – this is how you start.

If you've danced to the St. Bernard's waltz you'll remember where the '*stamp, stamp*' comes in the music. That's where you '*slap slap*' in this exercise!

Repeat this routine to take 16 bars in all – then just 'Rock' on your seat for the next 8 – and do the exercise once more to make up the complete 32 bars.

(Music: St. Bernard's Waltz – 8 bars)

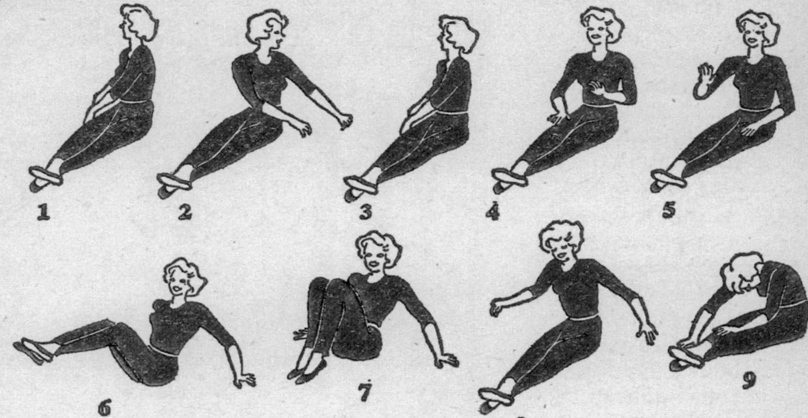


**1** Sit with ankles crossed – twist round to right. **2** Twist round to left, fingers tipping floor. **3** Twist round to right again. **4** Slap right knee with right hand. Sit tall. **5** Slap left knee with left hand.

**6** Lean back, uncross ankles, pulling knees up. **7** Tip floor with both feet on toes. **8** Cross ankles as you replace feet on floor. **9** Relax forward and slap floor with right hand. **10** Slap floor with left hand. Head down.

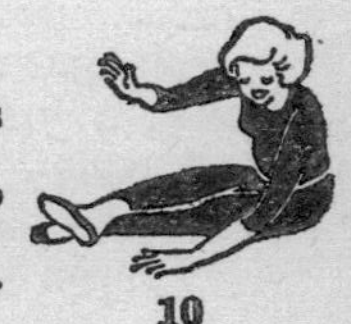

## **Sweep around** – a slimming movement giving grace and poise

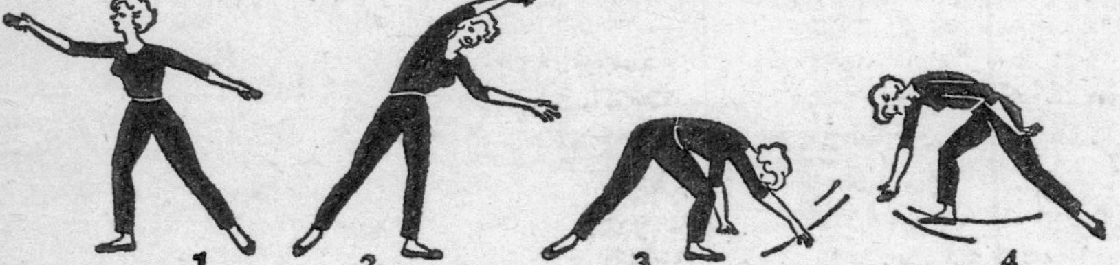


**1** Stretch out to right, weight on right foot, knees relaxed. **2** Rock weight on to left foot as right arm starts to circle.

**3** Continue circle by bending knees deeply and passing left foot. **4** Take weight across to right foot, hand just above floor.

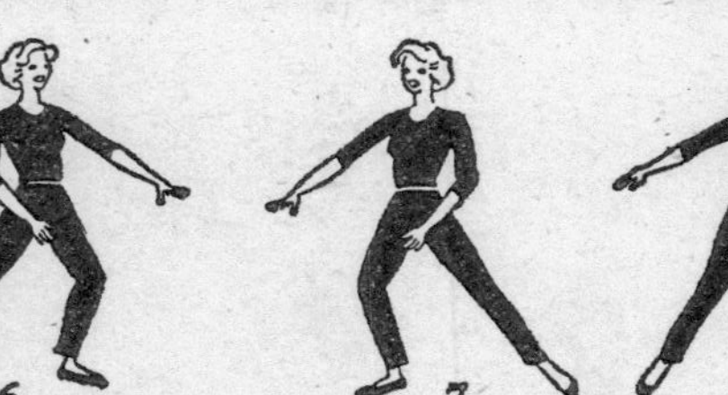


**5** Finish one complete circle by coming up again to starting position. **6** Rock to left with relaxed knees, arms following movement.

**7** Rock back on to right foot; rock left and stretch left arm out to begin again. (8)

Start right by having the weight on your right foot and stretching your right arm towards the wall. Sweep the arm from there across the ceiling to the left as you start your big circular movement. As you drop down to continue the circle, relax the head, knees bent deeply – sweep across in front of your feet and up again to where you started – drop the arm as you rock to left and right, then stretch out towards left – to begin again with the left arm.

(One sequence 8 bars of music. Repeat 4 times to 32-bar chorus.)

(Music: Slow foxtrot)